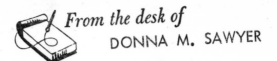

From the desk of
DONNA M. SAWYER

STROKE

STROKE

The Condition and the Patient

BY

JOHN E. SARNO, M.D.

*Associate Professor, Rehabilitation Medicine,
New York University School of Medicine, Director
Outpatient Services, Institute of Rehabilitation
Medicine, New York University Medical
Center, New York City*

AND

MARTHA TAYLOR SARNO, M.A.

*Assistant Professor, Clinical Rehabilitation Medicine,
New York University School of Medicine.
Director, Speech Pathology Services, Institute of
Rehabilitation Medicine, New York University
Medical Center, New York City*

INTRODUCTION BY HOWARD A. RUSK, M.D.

McGraw-Hill Book Company
New York   Toronto   London   Sydney

Library of Congress Catalog Card Number: 77–95830

ISBN 07–054739–4

345678910   VBVB   798765

Preface

In a sense, this book was written by those for whom it is primarily intended, the families and close friends of people who have had strokes. Most of the questions posed in these chapters have been asked by them countless times through the years so that this becomes a document of both their experience and ours—theirs in asking the questions and ours in answering them.

A catastrophic illness or injury invariably brings great physical and emotional turmoil to all those involved. If it is over quickly then all are restored to their former conditions. But if the illness or its residuals continue for long periods of time, as is often the case with stroke, and if it produces a change in the life pattern of the family, then the strains become severe and people become desperate for help.

The word *change* is the key. The patient sees himself as changed to something less than he was before and this is a blow to his ego, it erodes his self-confidence and causes him to withdraw and be depressed. Those close to him observe the changes in the patient's behavior and this disturbs and frightens them. Usually the way of life the family knew before is altered, more or less. Mother is not cooking and cleaning or Father can't work and the family income stops. Leisure patterns change, guests are not received as often—indeed, friends seem to shy away. Husbands or wives find themselves doing things they never expected to do—either for the patient or in the place of the patient.

To those who have had this experience or are having it at this moment, these words are no doubt painfully descriptive. Although the details vary, the quality of distress and anguish is common to all.

It is the purpose of this book to allay some of the fear, confusion and anxiety which attend a stroke. Over and over the patient's spouse has said, "I simply didn't know where to turn, what to do or whom to ask." No mere book can do what needs to be done in such a serious situation but we hope that it will provide a framework of information upon which can be built understanding and confidence.

Understanding is another key word. We believe that knowledge dispels fear and anxiety and that those who treat or work with stroke patients and their families have a major responsibility to help them understand the nature of stroke. Here again, this is not the total answer but it provides a basis upon which to build. As the personalities of people differ, so do their needs for information, guidance and support. The doctors, nurses and therapists who treat patients and talk to their families must be sensitive to these varying needs.

Because this is true and since this work is an outgrowth of direct contact with patients' families, we believe this book can be of value to all professionals who work with stroke patients. We have learned that rehabilitation medicine requires an extra dimension from those who work in the field. They must master the technical details of their specialties but must also learn the art of ministering to the emotional needs of patients and their families. This is no small task, for the problems are great.

Someone has said knowledge is power, and indeed there is great strength needed to overcome the difficulties which stroke brings. If this book can in some way contribute to that kind of power, we will consider the effort to produce it to have been worthwhile.

Contents

Introduction

Howard A. Rusk, M.D.

Stroke is a word that has always struck terror into the hearts of both patients and their families. Unfortunately, there are estimated to be more than two million victims in the United States. Stroke is one of the triumvirate with heart disease and cancer as the leading causes of death and disability.

In the past it was thought that after the first stroke you waited, usually in a wheelchair, rocking chair, back bedroom or nursing home for the second stroke to strike like lightning out of the blue. This would further disable you and then the third would be fatal. Imagine living with this anxiety and agony, like the sword of Damocles over your head night and day.

It is now well known that this is just not the fact. Individuals who recover from an initial stroke have an incidence of recurrence no different from others in the same age group who have never had a stroke. In talking with stroke patients and their families, I have found that this fact has been of immense comfort to them.

Stroke: The Condition and the Patient makes an invaluable contribution to the understanding of the problem and what can be done about it; understanding for the patient, understanding for the family, and understanding for the physician. Its theme song is *understanding*.

Too often after recovery from the initial insult, patients

are left to drift passively without sail or rudder. In analyzing the cause of stroke, physical consequences, speech disorders, the intellectual and emotional aspects, rehabilitation and prognosis, a guide to action in management is detailed. The book provides not only direction but a new depth of understanding that all too often has not previously existed.

The problems of socialization for the stroke patient are fundamental. He needs an ongoing structured program after discharge from the hospital or rehabilitation center and it should be provided at home or in an outpatient facility. Hopefully, the community will become more active in this phase of rehabilitation. Until it does we see it as our continuing responsibility to help the patient find a social milieu which is conducive to his recovery.

One important point that is brought out in the book has to do with the assessment of brain damage. Experience of the authors has established the fact that immediately after stroke the degree and permanence of brain damage cannot be accurately assessed. This is due to the fact that in the healing process there is continuing edema for several weeks, and the symptoms of brain damage may be due to edema and not permanent brain damage. For this reason it is impossible to make a true and final prognosis in the early stages.

Continuing therapy in stroke patients must be appraised on an individual basis. In some instances, improvement will continue not only for months but for years.

Dr. and Mrs. Sarno have made a real contribution to the total understanding and rehabilitation of the stroke patient. Their book is more than a description of the patient and his condition, more than a description of treatment; it is a document interlaced with human understanding, compassion and hope.

CHAPTER 1

The Cause of Stroke

1. What is a stroke?
2. What is hemiplegia?
3. Are apoplexy and stroke the same thing?
4. Are spasm and stroke the same?
5. Is it true that one side of the brain controls the opposite side of the body?
6. Is stroke caused by brain damage?
7. What causes a stroke?
8. What causes the clot (thrombosis) or hemorrhage which results in a stroke?
9. What is an embolus and how does it come about?
10. It is difficult to understand why a blocked blood vessel or a hemorrhage causes a stroke. What exactly happens?
11. What other condition can cause strokes?
12. Can a tumor cause a stroke?
13. Can low blood pressure cause a stroke?
14. Can a stroke be caused by a blow to the head or an auto accident?
15. What does the heart have to do with causing a stroke?
16. Is a stroke the same as a heart attack?
17. Do drinking, smoking, or coffee have anything to do with the cause of stroke?
18. Are strokes caused by overwork?

19. What is the effect of salt intake on the cause of stroke?
20. What is a massive stroke?
21. Is there such a thing as a light stroke?
22. Can a stroke be predicted or prevented?
23. Do people ever have trouble with speech before the stroke comes on?
24. Does a person act differently in the weeks preceding a stroke?
25. Is it possible to have a stroke on both sides?
26. How can someone have a stroke after having had a complete checkup just a few days before?
27. Do more men than women have strokes?
28. Do strokes only occur in older people?
29. Are doctors doing research on the prevention of stroke?

Introduction

Although this book is about the effects of stroke, we have included this chapter on cause for two reasons.

One of our primary aims is to remove the mystery about stroke because people usually fear what they don't understand. Even though a subject may be unpleasant or scary, somehow it isn't quite so frightening if we know something about it and you cannot really understand stroke without having some knowledge of its cause.

Secondly, it is our hope that these questions on cause will help people to understand what practical things can be done to prevent the conditions which lead to stroke. This is important for everyone since we are all interested in preventive medicine. It is important for the stroke patient in order to reduce the possibility of a second episode. We have found that people are more apt to be conscientious about following the doctor's recommendations if they understand the reasons for them.

1. What is a stroke?

It is an affliction of the brain which is sudden in onset and causes weakness of one side of the body and other possible symptoms such as loss of sensation, speech disturbance, visual difficulty, and intellectual or emotional disorders. Not all patients have all of these symptoms, but no matter how mild or severe it is, a stroke is an ordeal for the patient and his family. It is the purpose of this book to explain the disease and the problems it produces for the patient and those who are close to him.

A stroke is often referred to by doctors as a cerebral vascular accident or *hemiplegia*.

2. What is hemiplegia?

This word refers to the weakness which usually occurs on one side of the body or the other with a stroke. It is used a great deal among doctors and is almost synonymous with the term "stroke." For example, doctors will refer to patients with weakness on the left side as left hemiplegics and on the right as right hemiplegics. It is not entirely accurate to do this since there may be symptoms other than weakness on the affected side of the body. But in medicine, as in other fields, words are often used out of habit or custom even though they may not be entirely accurate.

The origin of the word is interesting; it is from the Greek. *Hemi* means half and *plegia* means paralysis. Again, it is often used inaccurately in another way since most patients are not paralyzed but only weak on one side.

3. Are apoplexy and stroke the same thing?

The words "apoplexy" and "stroke" have no real medical meaning, but both refer to the same thing—the sudden onset of a vascular accident in the brain. Apoplexy is rarely used any more, but the word "stroke" has become thoroughly entrenched in the English language.

4. Are spasm and stroke the same?

The term "spasm" is used a great deal in medicine, but whether such a thing occurs is a matter for debate. What is referred to as a spasm is not the same thing as a stroke.

When someone has temporary symptoms of stroke which last only minutes to hours, he is often said to have had a spasm. These symptoms are described in detail later in this chapter. They are temporary because the blood vessel in the brain is not closed off completely but is only smaller in diameter, reducing the blood flow to a part of the brain for a short time but never shutting it off completely.

What this means will perhaps be clearer after the next few answers. The point of this answer is that spasm and stroke are not the same thing.

5. Is it true that one side of the brain controls the opposite side of the body?

The brain is a fascinating and complicated organ having many important functions. Among these are the control of all body movements and the interpretation of sensations from all parts of the body, including things seen, heard, and smelled. It contains the centers for language, thinking, and emotion.

Many of these functions are shared by both sides of the brain, but it is perfectly true that with some of them one-half of the brain controls the opposite side of the body. For example, if the left half of the brain is damaged by a stroke, movement of the right arm, right leg, and right side of the face can be disturbed; sensation on the right side of the body may not be normal; and the peripheral field of vision on the right may be lost. Not all of these things occur with every stroke.

Hearing is interpreted on both sides of the brain from both ears. Hence, hearing is not damaged with a stroke.

There is only one important human activity which is exclusively the responsibility of one side of the brain and that is *speech*. In the majority of people the speech centers are on the left side of the brain. It is for this reason that a stroke involving the left hemisphere and causing weakness to the right side of the body (right hemiplegia) may also produce a speech disturbance. Chapter 3 gives detailed information on speech disorders.

6. Is stroke caused by brain damage?

It is more accurate to say that brain damage is caused by stroke. In other words, stroke refers to the sudden deprivation of some part of the brain of its blood supply, and as a result this portion of the brain is damaged. The important thing to remember is that nature can often repair the damage.

7. What causes a stroke?

In the days following the onset of a stroke this question may occur over and over in the minds of the patient and those close to him. They are haunted by a persistently recurrent "Why?" and often by the more poignant and painful "Why me?" Some know that hypertension (high blood pressure) has something to do with it or that hardening of the arteries (arteriosclerosis or atherosclerosis) may be involved, but it is rare to find someone who has a comprehensive understanding of the factors which lead to a cerebral vascular accident.

In general, the desire to understand the cause of stroke stems from still another question: "What did I do wrong?" A wife or husband feels guilty for not having insisted that the patient have a checkup or stop working so hard. Those close to the patient ask themselves whether *they* did anything to precipitate the attack, and many patients or families wonder if it was punishment for wrongdoing. There are many such reactions.

An equally important reason why people want to understand the cause of stroke is their desire to prevent another one. One can do nothing about what might have been—but sometimes significant things can be done to prevent a recurrence. These will be pointed out as we go along.

The following explanation represents our own views on the cause of stroke. What is presented as fact is medically accepted, but there are certain factors which have not as yet been proved according to the scientific method and which can be given only as theory or opinion. We shall identify what is fact, what is theory, and what is opinion.

It may be shocking but it is probably true that the process which culminates in a stroke starts thirty to forty years before the stroke occurs. (See Question 8.) The actual "apoplectic" episode, which causes the sudden loss of consciousness, paralysis of an arm and leg, speech disorder, or any of the other possible consequences of a stroke, results from a sudden deprivation of some part of the brain of its blood supply and therefore of its nutrient and oxygen supply. It is common knowledge that all body tissues need oxygen to survive, and that oxygen is brought to tissues in the blood through blood vessels (arteries). What happens with stroke is a sudden interference with this system, most commonly in one of three ways: (1) a clot forms in an artery; (2) the wall of an artery ruptures and causes a hemorrhage (bleeding); or (3) a piece of a clot, having formed elsewhere in the body, breaks loose, travels to the brain, and plugs a blood vessel.

7

Any of these three occurrences is known as a cerebral vascular accident. The first is more properly called a *cerebral thrombosis,* the second a *cerebral hemorrhage,* and the third a *cerebral embolism.*

Since each of the vessels in the brain supplies blood to a particular part of the brain, sudden plugging of an artery means that the brain tissue it serves is immediately deprived of most of its blood supply. (We say "most" because the body has emergency systems which we shall later describe.) Sudden plugging is the process which occurs with thrombosis or embolism.

In the case of hemorrhage, the situation is considerably different and usually more severe since a large proportion of hemorrhages cause death. Here blood escapes through a weak spot in the blood vessel wall and damages brain tissue by compression. In addition, the area of brain supplied by the ruptured artery may receive an insufficient supply of blood causing further damage to brain cells.

It is likely that strokes would produce even more damage than they do were it not for the existence of a kind of emergency system of blood vessels. When something happens to close off an artery anywhere in the body, nature attempts to get more blood to the tissues supplied by that artery to make up for the reduced flow of blood. It does this by making use of auxiliary vessels which go to the same area. If the process of occlusion is slow enough, these auxiliary vessels have an opportunity to enlarge, and sometimes they may actually provide the entire blood supply for a part of the brain. This has been observed on X-ray studies where, although the main artery to a portion of the brain has closed off completely, a stroke does not occur because the auxiliaries have grown large enough to supply the area adequately.

Even if the closure of a vessel is sudden, as with an embolism, there are other channels to the same part of the brain which bring in blood and reduce the amount of damage done.

This is the way of nature—to heal, to make compensations or substitutions in order to keep the body functioning. Of course, nature does not always work rapidly and thoroughly enough or there would be fewer strokes—and there would be no aging process. But it is likely that the severity of some strokes is reduced because of these collateral blood vessels.

8. What causes the clot (thrombosis) or hemorrhage which results in a stroke?

Relatively early in life the process commonly known as hardening of the arteries begins to take place. It is more properly known as *arteriosclerosis* or *atherosclerosis*. We know it occurs quite early since postmortem examinations on young men killed in battle or accidents have revealed the presence of atherosclerotic deposits in the walls of blood vessels. As one grows older these deposits increase both in number and size, and eventually there may be such a large accumulation at one point in a blood vessel that a blood clot forms, increases in size, and then occludes the artery. Another possibility is that the artery ruptures at the site of a large arteriosclerotic deposit, and the patient suffers a hemorrhage.

Now, if one is to prevent thrombosis or hemorrhage, the obvious question is "How can you prevent arteriosclerosis?" or better "What causes arteriosclerosis?" Unfortunately, we do not yet know the precise answers to these questions, but research has begun to throw some light on the subject.

It is undoubtedly true that arteriosclerosis is part of the aging process. But we believe that the rate at which it develops is affected by five important things: diet, exercise, blood pressure, nervous tension, and heredity. There are no doubt many other factors which influence the development

9

of atherosclerotic deposits, but we know even less about them than we do about the five named.

DIET: At the present time intensive investigation is going on to determine what role cholesterol plays in this problem, and a great deal of effort is being devoted to a search for a medication which will reduce cholesterol in the blood. Since cholesterol is present in some foods, it is natural to wonder how important diet is.

It is known that cholesterol crystals are deposited in the walls of arteries and that this tends to occur more in certain arteries than in others, but why they are deposited, how important the amount of cholesterol in the blood is, what factors account for the level of blood cholesterol, and many other questions are still unanswered. It is also possible that other blood substances contribute to arteriosclerosis.

Whatever the role of these substances, one thing seems clear: overeating and overweight have a lot to do with arteriosclerosis. What is the evidence for this? Besides stroke, certain heart attacks are caused by arteriosclerosis. During World War II the incidence of heart attacks and strokes in England and Germany, two countries from which statistics are available, went way down. Both countries had a scarcity of food during the war, and both had a decrease in the number of strokes and heart attacks. It is hard to escape the conclusion that eating less was at least partially responsible for this.

It is known that being overweight may also contribute to high blood pressure and, as we shall see in a moment, an elevated pressure probably increases hardening of the arteries. There are, then, two good reasons why weight should be reduced if it is high, or kept low: to slow down arteriosclerosis and to help prevent hypertension. It is just as important for someone who has had a stroke to go on a diet as for someone who is trying to prevent one.

Something else which should be mentioned here is that people with *diabetes* tend to develop arteriosclerosis more rapidly. It is well known that the diabetes of later life most often occurs in people who are overweight. Here, then, is an additional piece of evidence that excessive food intake hastens arteriosclerosis.

EXERCISE: It was just stated that the lack of food was probably good for the British and Germans during the war, at least with regard to heart attacks and strokes. But it may be that an increase in physical activity was also beneficial. This is one of those facts which has not been proved, but it is our belief that the human body was designed for vigorous activity and that exercise probably slows down the rate of hardening of the arteries. After a stroke, patients usually exercise a great deal as part of the rehabilitation process. Unless there are other medical conditions which prohibit exercise, we urge all of our patients to be as active as possible.

BLOOD PRESSURE: High blood pressure, or hypertension as it is known to doctors, is another medical mystery which is slowly being solved. From the evidence at hand, it seems that hypertension increases the rate of arteriosclerotic deposits. It probably also increases the chances that a blood vessel will rupture at a weak spot.

It is likely that many things tend to produce hypertension; among them, overweight, nervous tension, perhaps specific substances like salt. It is believed that the kidney plays an important role in pressure regulation, and a number of kidney diseases are associated with a rise in blood pressure. The subject is a complicated one and cannot be detailed here.

What is important is that high blood pressure should always be treated, before or after a stroke, and one must pay attention to the factors which can make it worse like over-weight and nervous tension.

NERVOUS TENSION: Of the five factors mentioned this is the most difficult to pin down. We strongly suspect that tension contributes to high blood pressure and perhaps to the speed of the arteriosclerotic process, but this has not been proved. However, we need not wait for the proof—the suspicion is enough.

Tension-producing situations must be avoided by some-one who has had a stroke. Returning to a high-pressure job is obviously unwise. This is discussed more thoroughly in Question 37, Chapter 4.

HEREDITY: Unfortunately, we cannot choose our ancestors, and the practical implication of this is that there are people who seem to be born with certain tendencies. Some have high cholesterol levels in the blood despite diets low in choles-terol, others naturally tend to be overweight, and there are those who seem to develop arteriosclerosis at an unusually early age. Though such problems are still poorly under-stood, there is no doubt that eventually ways will be found to counteract them.

As we can see, the factors that contribute to arterioscle-rosis are related to each other. Overweight predisposes to hardening of the arteries and hypertension; hypertension increases arteriosclerosis and the possibility of hemorrhage; the lack of exercise makes weight gain easier and keeps nervous tension bottled up within; tension may cause over-eating and contribute to high blood pressure. Together they are part of a biological riddle which medical science is try-ing to solve. A great deal has been learned already, treat-ment methods are vastly improved, and the future looks bright.

9. What is an embolus and how does it come about?

This is the third major cause of stroke and the least common. An *embolus* is a more or less solid piece of matter which travels in the blood stream and eventually gets stuck in a blood vessel, thereby cutting off the flow of blood to the tissue which that artery supplies. It can happen in a number of places in the body, and when it occurs in the brain it causes a stroke.

In these cases the embolus is a portion of a clot which previously formed in the heart or large blood vessels leading from the heart. Unlike a thrombosis, there is usually no warning.

On the other hand, doctors often know when the danger of an embolus exists and do everything they can to prevent it. In most cases there is some preexisting heart condition which favors the formation of a clot on a valve or on one of the inside walls of the heart.

A stroke caused by an embolus usually looks no different from one caused by a thrombosis or hemorrhage and the outcome is just as varied.

10. It is difficult to understand why a blocked blood vessel or a hemorrhage causes a stroke. What exactly happens?

Basically, it is the lack of oxygen which causes the stroke since the absence of oxygen produces damage to brain cells. If this happened to cells of the skin, the tissue would slough off and there would be an ulcer. In terms of body function this would mean that part of the body's protective covering, the skin, would be lost, and it would be possible for foreign substances like dirt or bacteria to enter the body. In other organs different kinds of function are disturbed by damaged tissue—an impaired kidney cannot produce urine, a damaged heart cannot pump blood as well.

Brain cells have many important functions. A lack of oxygen suddenly interferes with some of them: the arm and leg on one side may become paralyzed; normal sensation or the peripheral vision on that side may be diminished; there may be weakness of the facial muscles and perhaps a speech disturbance.

What precisely happens depends on which side of the brain is involved, and where on that side the damage has occurred. The left side of the brain (left hemisphere) controls the right side of the body and vice versa. Also of extreme importance, the left hemisphere usually contains the centers for language or communication.

In subsequent chapters the physical, intellectual, emotional, and speech consequences of stroke will be described. There is great variation from patient to patient because the same precise area of the brain is not involved in each person. What each case has in common, however, is the temporary or permanent interference with one or more vital brain functions as a result of the lack of oxygen.

11. What other conditions can cause strokes?

Although most of the conditions have already been mentioned, there are a few others which one may hear about. They are all less common than those caused by clotting or hemorrhage due to arteriosclerosis and high blood pressure, and some are rare.

1. Some people are born with a weak spot along the course of an artery in the brain (*aneurysm*). For reasons not well understood the spot may begin to balloon out, much like a weak spot on a tire, and as it does so it begins to compress tissue. If it compresses another blood vessel, the patient may

begin to have the early signs of stroke; if it occludes an artery completely, the patient has a complete stroke. Even more serious, there may be a blowout with hemorrhage into brain tissue. Fortunately, these conditions can be detected by X-ray, and surgeons are becoming more and more skilled at dealing with them.

2. A localized infection within brain tissue (called an *abscess*) can cause a stroke-like picture by compression. If it is discovered and promptly treated, the patient can have good recovery.

3. Bacterial infections in the heart sometimes cause clots to form which then embolize to the brain.

4. Syphilis can damage the walls of arteries in the brain and lead to stroke.

5. Meningitis may cause narrowing of brain arteries and thereby create the possibility of clot formation.

6. Leukemia has been known to cause stroke by damaging blood vessels in the brain.

7. Encephalitis is a more generalized infection in the brain and may cause symptoms that look like a stroke.

12. Can a tumor cause a stroke?

There are many types of brain tumor, but something they all have in common is that they take up space and compress some part of the brain. Since all of the brain is vital to normal body function, compression of even small areas will usually produce symptoms. For example, an arm may become weak, the eyes may not move correctly, or speech may be impaired.

Although there are some important differences in the symptoms produced, a tumor may cause changes in the patient which look like a stroke. The biggest difference is that a tumor usually takes months or years to develop, and a stroke occurs in minutes or hours and, rarely, over a period of

15

days. If the tumor happens to compress a vital blood vessel all of a sudden, the patient may look as though he has had the usual kind of stroke.

The important thing to bear in mind is that there are many things which cause stroke, and the specialist in diseases of the nervous system, the neurologist, should always be consulted so that the precise cause can be determined.

13. Can low blood pressure cause a stroke?

The low blood pressure that most people talk about does not cause stroke. One often hears someone say that he has just had his blood pressure checked and it is low. This means low in comparison to average or high blood pressure, but it does not imply that low pressure is abnormal or dangerous. As a matter of fact it is generally a good thing to have low blood pressure.

Although what has been said above is generally true, there are occasional situations when the doctor wants the patient's blood pressure to be higher. These are quite rare, and the average person need not be concerned about them.

14. Can a stroke be caused by a blow to the head or an auto accident?

Strictly speaking, no, since by stroke we usually mean a vascular accident in the brain occurring as a result of a thrombosis, a hemorrhage, or an embolism. However, a blow to the head can cause symptoms similar to those seen in the usual stroke. The major reason for this is the hemorrhage in the brain which often follows a blow, although there may be damage to tissue without bleeding.

As might be expected, a head injury can affect any of the systems described before: motor, sensory, language, visual, intellectual, or emotional. Therefore, although the patterns of involvement are usually different from those of a typical stroke, many of the things said in this book apply to head injuries.

15. What does the heart have to do with causing a stroke?

The great majority of people with heart conditions need not fear connection with stroke. Very few strokes are caused by heart disease, and it is rare for heart conditions to complicate the neurological problems of someone who has already had a stroke.

Someone with *heart failure* may actually do better after a stroke since high blood pressure usually returns to normal with a stroke, easing the strain on the heart. In turn, this permits the heart to do its job more efficiently, which includes sending an adequate blood supply to the brain.

Another common heart condition—*coronary thrombosis*—similarly is not related to the onset of stroke except in the rare cases described below.

The most important relationship between a cardiac condition and stroke exists when someone develops a clot (*thrombosis*) within one of the chambers of the heart. Most commonly the thrombosis forms on a diseased heart valve, usually the result of rheumatic fever. It may also form on a valve which is defective from birth. Less commonly, it can form on the inside wall of a heart chamber which is beating abnormally.

In all of these cases nothing will happen unless a piece of the clot breaks loose, travels in the blood stream to the brain, and blocks a blood vessel there. This can often be prevented by the use of appropriate medications. If it occurs, the patient is said to have had a stroke due to an embolus. Thus, a small number of strokes are actually caused by heart disease.

For the most part, however, heart disease does not cause strokes, and strokes do not cause cardiac conditions or make them worse.

16. Is a stroke the same as a heart attack?

Stroke refers only to vascular accident in the brain. The same type of occurrence in the heart is called a coronary occlusion, coronary thrombosis, or myocardial infarction.

17. Do drinking, smoking, or coffee have anything to do with the cause of stroke?

There is no evidence that drinking alcoholic beverages in moderation contributes to stroke. It is likely that the relaxation and good feelings induced by a social drink are actually beneficial. However, since heavy drinking can contribute to overweight, it may be an indirect factor in the causation of stroke.

But what about coffee, the great American elixir without which most people can't (so they think) start the day, which is required for periodic sustenance as they wrestle with the daily affairs of life, and which is often the last indulgence before turning out the light at night. We are told that Americans consume astronomic quantities of coffee each day and with it significant amounts of caffeine. The great French writer Balzac is said to have drunk himself to death —with coffee.

It has not been established as fact, but there is a suspicion that caffeine is not good for the cardiovascular system (heart and blood vessels). Therefore, it would seem that moderation in coffee drinking might be wise—just in case caffeine has something to do with high blood pressure, arteriosclerosis, or both.

In the matter of smoking, the evidence has been steadily accumulating that this habit is definitely bad for the cardiovascular system. It is quite clear that certain forms of heart disease are more common in smokers, and, by extension, one would expect that the blood vessels of the brain might be adversely affected by nicotine.

With this in mind it is probably accurate to say that smoking contributes to the conditions which precede stroke. One must therefore ask himself whether the pleasure of smoking is worth its potential dangers. Certainly people who have had the signs of an impending stroke or have actually had one ought not to smoke.

18. Are strokes caused by overwork?

Not by overwork alone. Earlier in this chapter we described in some detail how strokes occur and what causes them. Hardening of the arteries, high blood pressure, overweight, underexercise, excessive tension, heredity, excessive caffeine or nicotine—all play a role of greater or lesser significance.

When long hours of very hard work contribute to nervous tension, poor eating habits, insufficient sleep, or excessive use of coffee and cigarettes, then indeed they may contribute to the onset of a stroke. Some people thrive on work, however, and are healthiest and happiest when they're hard at it. What makes the difference is whether a person suffers from too much work or whether he thrives on it.

19. What is the effect of salt intake on the cause of stroke?

A number of years ago medical scientists suggested a relationship between salt in the diet and high blood pressure. As a result, patients with hypertension were often placed on a diet which was extremely low in salt, and many of them had significant reductions in blood pressure. These diets are rarely prescribed anymore.

In the present treatment of hypertension it is almost routine to give one of a class of medications which allows the kidney to excrete more salt than it ordinarily would. Under this method of treatment the salt in the body is kept down by increasing the amount of excretion rather than limiting the amount of intake.

This is related to stroke because high blood pressure is one of the factors which seems to predispose to stroke. By keeping the pressure down, one may be reducing the possibility of a stroke.

20. What is a massive stroke?

This simply refers to one in which a great deal of damage has been done. In such cases the arm and leg paralysis may be complete and all sensation on one side gone; there may be loss of peripheral vision on the affected side, a severe language disorder if the dominant side of the brain is involved, and intellectual and emotional problems.

However, it is important to know that a massive stroke does not necessarily mean permanent severe damage. Such patients can recover. What is of greater importance than the number and severity of symptoms immediately after the stroke is the actual cause of it. This will determine whether anything can be done surgically or the extent to which nature can heal the damaged tissue.

Parts of Chapter 6 deal with the process of healing and may be consulted for further information.

21. Is there such a thing as a light stroke?

Indeed there is, and many strokes are light. It means that the clot or hemorrhage or embolus was small, that less brain tissue was injured, and, therefore, that the patient had fewer symptoms.

Patients with light strokes usually recover fully or have very little residual disability.

22. Can a stroke be predicted or prevented?

Although we are primarily concerned in this book with the person who has already had a stroke, this question is included because it is asked so often and because the answer may be of importance in preventing further trouble.

Some of the basic causes of stroke have already been described, and it has been suggested that high blood pressure, overweight, and excessive nervous tension should be controlled. These are long-term matters, however, and apply to all of us, whether or not we have had a stroke.

Now let us be more specific and see how a stroke can be prevented in someone who is a possible candidate. Prediction or prevention depends on the following:

1. The recognition of symptoms which precede an outright stroke.

2. The identification of the place in the body where the trouble is located and the kind of trouble which is developing.

3. The ability to do something about the problem before a stroke occurs.

1. SYMPTOMS: The commonest ones will be described, but we should first point out that some of these symptoms can be caused by other conditions, and one who observes them should not assume that a stroke is coming. They are usually temporary or transient, lasting from a few seconds to a few days. In all cases a doctor should be consulted so that a proper investigation can be done to determine the exact cause of the symptom. Here is a list:

a. Dizziness. This may occur with or without a change in body position. For example, sometimes a person gets dizzy only upon getting out of bed. Dizziness is so common in people of all ages we almost hesitate to put it on the list except that it may be a sign of an impending stroke.

21

b. Weakness of the arm, hand, or leg on one or both sides of the body. Since the trouble spot in the circulation to the brain varies from patient to patient any combination of weakness can occur, although it is most likely to be the arm and leg on one side.

c. Weakness of the facial muscles with sagging on one side or the other.

d. Feelings of numbness or "tingling" in an arm or leg; inability to feel painful or very warm things. These are indicative of a disturbance in the sensory system and will be described in greater detail in Chapter 2.

e. Cramps in an arm with exercise; coldness or pain in the fingers.

f. Clumsiness in the use of a hand or a mild balance problem.

g. A speech problem—any of those described in Chapter 3 but usually in a very mild form. This includes aphasia, peripheral dysarthria, and cortical dysarthria.

h. Visual disturbances—this may be a temporary loss of vision in one eye or the other or just the loss of the so-called peripheral field, which is what one sees out of the "side of the eyes" when looking straight ahead.

i. Forgetfulness or some other mild problem with the thinking mechanism.

j. Undue flushing of the face. This may be indicative of a sudden rise in blood pressure or the existence of a rare condition in which there are too many red cells in the blood.

2 & 3: TYPE AND LOCATION OF THE TROUBLE AND WHAT CAN BE DONE ABOUT IT

a. If one thinks of the cells of the brain as though they were leaves on a tree, one can imagine how blood gets to them. It starts out in the trunk, which is like the great vessel

that comes out of the top of the heart, branches off in
one of a few main branches, smaller than the trunk bu
still very large, then to smaller and smaller branches unt
it gets to each leaf. The leaves are like the cells in th
brain. Anything that interferes with the circulatic
through any of these branches on the way to brain cel
can deprive them of oxygen and nourishment and ca
cause some of the symptoms just described.

Now let us be more specific. Blockage in the main trun
(aorta) is rarely the cause of stroke. However, it is est
mated that around 35 percent of all strokes may be cause
by an obstruction in one of the large arteries which branc
off the main trunk. Therefore, transient symptoms may b
a sign that one of these blood vessels is becomin
obstructed by arteriosclerosis. There are a number c
tests which can be done by the doctor to find out if ther
is serious narrowing in one of these arteries, both by phys
ical examination and special X-ray techniques. If this i
found, depending on the exact location and the extent c
the narrowing, surgery may be done either to remove th
section of narrowed artery or to bypass it with a graft. I
the latter case, one actually makes a new channe
attached to the healthy portions of the vessel above an
below the site of obstruction; either a synthetic materia
like Dacron or a piece of one of the patient's own vein
can be used.

It should be clear that these large arteries upon whicl
surgery may be performed are located outside of the hea
(in the chest or neck) and therefore can be reached. Th
smaller branches within the brain itself cannot be oper
ated upon in this fashion.

b. Now let us suppose that a patient is beginning to have
symptoms or perhaps even a "little stroke," but that the
site of obstruction appears to be in one of the smalle
arteries in the brain itself. Although they are smaller than

23

the branches in the chest and neck, these arteries may be very important and complete occlusion can result in a full-blown stroke. What does one do in this case?

Although there is some difference of opinion about the effectiveness of this procedure, many doctors employ drugs which will make the blood "thinner" in an effort to prevent a clot from forming at the site of partial obstruction. Remember that arteriosclerotic deposits in the wall of the artery have made the channel narrower, which in turn makes it more likely that a clot will begin to form at this location. Blood-thinning drugs are used to prevent this from happening.

If this same patient has high blood pressure, it may also be desirable to treat this. The doctor must bear in mind, however, that a large reduction in blood pressure may further reduce blood supply to the area of the brain involved, and so he usually approaches this treatment very carefully.

c. Recall that one must know what is liable to cause a stroke in order to try to prevent it. There are situations in which disease of the heart may be the precipitating factor. Rheumatic fever, which occurs in children and young people, often does permanent damage to one or more of the valves of the heart. These scarred valves seem to favor the formation of clots, and once a clot is formed, a piece may break off, travel to the brain, and plug an artery, as described earlier. Prevention of these valve clots by drugs or surgery can be important in stroke prevention.

Other conditions also favor the formation of clots within the chambers of the heart. In every case it is important that all heart ailments be carefully treated.

d. We have mentioned the blood condition in which there is an excess of red cells. This makes the blood thicker and more liable to clot and can be treated by bleeding the

patient (as barbers used to do) or destroying some of these cells with appropriate drugs. Fortunately, this is a very rare condition.

In summary, some strokes can be prevented. It requires good luck, awareness of the warning signs, and prompt, appropriate treatment. With each day that passes the medical profession learns more about these matters and in consequence becomes better able to prevent both new and recurrent strokes.

23. Do people ever have trouble with speech before the stroke comes on?

In the preceding answer, it was pointed out that some patients are warned of an impending stroke by the appearance of mild symptoms that may include problems with speech. A wife may notice that her husband hesitates while speaking or doesn't seem to understand everything that's said to him. In fact, any of the stroke symptoms described in this book can be seen before the stroke occurs, and when they are, a doctor should be consulted immediately.

24. Does a person act differently in the weeks preceding a stroke?

Two men who have written books about their strokes, Eric Hodgins and Guy Wint, both say that they were very depressed for many weeks preceding their strokes. It is doubtful that this is a universal symptom, however, for many strokes come on without any warning such as this. Furthermore, it may have been coincidence in these two writers although the same thing has been described by other patients.

Depression is a very common symptom in all kinds of people, and it should not be assumed that it always precedes a stroke. However, if this symptom is found along with others, it is wise to check with the doctor.

25. Is it possible to have a stroke on both sides?

If this question refers to a stroke on both sides *at the same time,* the possibilities are very slim. This is so rare that many doctors never see such a patient, and in rehabilitation centers where many people with stroke come for treatment, it is quite unusual.

It is possible for a patient to have a stroke on both sides *at different times.* By far the largest group of patients consists of those who have involvement of only one side of the brain and therefore only one side of the body.

26. How can someone have a stroke after having had a complete checkup just a few days before?

This is a question which is asked frequently because it is very frightening and perplexing when it happens.

The reason is that there is really no way to predict a stroke unless one is having some of the premonitory symptoms discussed in Questions 22 and 23. On the other hand, we must face the fact that many people are candidates for stroke by virtue of age, general physical condition, etc. In Question 7 we stated that most strokes are thirty to forty years in the making. This means that the majority of them are a result of the aging process, and there is little one can do to prevent them.

With regard to medical examinations, even when these are very thorough, there is a limit to what can be detected. The human body is not a machine; it is a dynamic, changing mechanism of great complexity, and it is impossible to know everything about its function even with a good examination.

As we approach old age we must be prepared for the unexpected. This is surely not a comforting thought, but it is a part of life and must be accepted even as we accept its pleasures and its joys.

27. Do more men than women have strokes?

Yes. Roughly, twice as many men have strokes. The reasons are not entirely clear but are undoubtedly related to the incidence of arteriosclerosis and hypertension in men as contrasted with women.

Hormones may play a part in this since women tend to have far fewer strokes before menopause. This is so striking that there has been some research into the idea of having men take female hormones to prevent stroke. So far it has not been successful since the hormones (estrogens) cause undesirable effects such as loss of the sexual urge and enlargement of breast tissue.

28. Do strokes only occur in older people?

Strokes occur more often in older people but not exclusively. This is because the majority of strokes result from the gradual accumulation of arteriosclerotic deposits in blood vessels (arteries), and it takes many years for these to build up. In the unfortunate few who tend to develop hardening of the arteries at an early age, a stroke may occur in middle age.

In previous answers in this chapter other causes of stroke have been mentioned, some of which may precipitate an attack in younger people. An aneurysm (the weak spot in the wall of an artery) may rupture in a relatively young person. People with trouble on the valves of the heart due to rheumatic fever or congenital deformities may form clots which travel to the brain and plug a vessel. The condition called *polycythemia* (an increase in the number of red blood cells), which was described as a cause, may occur in young people. Fortunately, these are very rare and account for a small percentage of the total number of strokes which occur.

29. Are doctors doing research on the prevention of stroke?

The fight to prevent stroke is proceeding on many fronts.

For example, there is research into the causes of arteriosclerosis, which means that there are studies being done on the metabolism of cholesterol, the causes and treatment of high blood pressure and diabetes, how and why blood clots form and how to prevent them, whether smoking contributes to arteriosclerosis, and if and how tension and obesity hasten the process. The idea behind all of these efforts is that the more we know about the causes of a condition, the more likely we are to be able to prevent it.

Research is also being done on the prevention of hardening of the arteries through the use of drugs and through diet.

Prevention of the stroke itself is a matter of detecting narrowed blood vessels and relieving obstructions, and many doctors are working on better means of doing these two things.

It is common knowledge that the Federal government through many of its health agencies is an active participant in the effort to prevent stroke. It is reassuring to know that the scientific and financial resources of the government are also committed to the solution of this great problem.

CHAPTER 2

~~~~~~

The Physical Consequences of Stroke

1. How does a stroke cause weakness or paralysis on one side of the body?
2. Can a stroke cause loss of sensation in parts of the body?
3. How may a stroke affect vision?
4. Why do some patients have jerky movements of the arm and leg after a stroke?
5. Does a stroke affect hearing or smell?
6. Does a stroke affect the functioning of internal organs?
7. What does handedness have to do with a stroke?
8. What do you notice when you look at someone who has had a stroke?
9. Can you describe the physical changes which occur right after a stroke and how they recover?
10. Can a person have involvement of both sides of the body after a stroke?
11. How does the doctor decide how much damage the stroke did?
12. What tests are done after someone has had a stroke?
13. What is spasticity?

14. Why does the patient's paralyzed arm move when he yawns? Does it mean the arm is getting better?
15. Why does the patient's arm stiffen when he walks?
16. Why is it that sometimes a person's leg will get better but not his arm?
17. Why is the patient not able to use his hand very well even though he has good strength in it?
18. Why is the patient's balance poor when he first begins to walk?
19. Why is the patient afraid of falling?
20. Why is the patient so tired?
21. Should the patient have extra rest every day?
22. Does a patient's sleep pattern change after a stroke?
23. Why does the stroke patient stop smoking?
24. Do the patient's tastes in food and drink change?
25. What does pain in the hemiplegic arm mean?
26. Why do some patients have trouble controlling bladder and bowel function after a stroke?
27. What happens to the blood pressure after a stroke?
28. What is a seizure?
29. Do seizures have anything to do with stroke?
30. Does a stroke affect the wearing of dentures?
31. Why does the patient's voice sometimes change in pitch after a stroke?

Introduction

A stroke may cause changes in a number of different functions. This is because the brain is such an important part of the human body. In a sense it is like the power station that provides electricity for the lights, appliances, machinery, etc., which are so essential for life in a modern society.

But the brain is much more than a power station. It controls movements of the arms and legs, in fact, of all the outer muscles of the body; it makes sense out of everything the skin feels, the eyes see, the ears hear, and the nose smells. It thinks, remembers, imagines; it directs us to laugh or cry, run away or fight, be angry or loving. The brain is what makes us the very special animals that we are: "a little lower than the angels" and considerably higher than the apes.

This chapter deals with some of those aspects of brain function which we have in common with the lower animals. They include controlling body movements, interpreting body sensations, interpreting vision, interpreting hearing, controlling internal organs, and interpreting smell.

We shall describe how the brain does its job in each case and then show how a stroke may interfere with these functions.

1. How does a stroke cause weakness or paralysis on one side of the body?

One of the most important brain functions is the control of body movements. Let us imagine that Mr. A has decided

31

to get up and flip the dial on his television set—he is tired of the baseball game and wants to watch a horse race. Having made the decision, he puts his beer down on the end table, puts his hands on the arms of his easy chair, hoists his body out of the chair, and takes some steps toward the television set. Each one of these movements required the coordination (cooperation) of dozens of muscles in his arms, legs, and body, and all of them received their initial directions from one particular part of the brain. Once these orders were sent out from the movement center, other parts of the brain helped to make the movements smooth, and messages went back from the arms and legs to the brain (electronics engineers call this *feedback*) to make sure that the movements stayed smooth. We perform thousands of acts like these each day and never realize that each of us has a magnificent computer in his head which makes them possible.

The brain is divided into two halves (hemispheres), and for some reason that is not entirely clear, nature arranged things so that the left side of the brain controls movement on the right side of the body and vice versa. Therefore, a stroke which involves the left half of the brain will affect the movements of the right side of the body—the right side of the face, the right arm and leg, the muscles on the right side of the neck, chest, and abdomen.

In the previous chapter the cause and actual mechanism of a stroke were described. It was pointed out that something interferes with the blood supply to a particular part of the brain, and as a consequence that part is damaged. When a person who has sustained a stroke loses the ability to move the right arm and leg, normally it means that some part of the left half of the brain has been damaged and that the messages intended for the right arm and leg are not getting through. That, in essence, is what we mean when we say that an arm or leg has become weak or paralyzed—that the brain's message is not getting through. This is often called *hemi-*

plegia, which means paralysis of one half of the body (*hemi,* half; *plegia,* paralysis). (See Figure 2-1.)

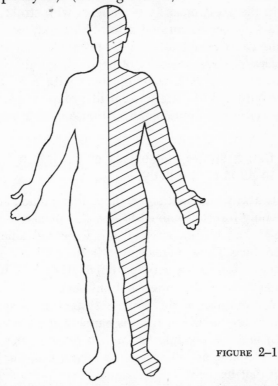

FIGURE 2–1

In order to better understand the kind of weakness which the stroke patient has, we must explain one more thing. It makes a difference where the wire has been cut. In the case of an electric power failure, it doesn't matter if the wire is cut at the power station or 1 foot away from the lamp—the light goes out. With the human nervous system, if the connection is cut in the brain the result is *spastic weakness,* and if it is cut close to the muscle it is called *flaccid weakness.* With spastic weakness the muscle does not shrink in size but may become very stiff and rigid so that it is difficult even for someone else to move the patient's arm. This *spasticity* is often a problem, and it will be discussed more fully in the answers to later questions.

In the great majority of patients with stroke, paralysis or weakness occurs on one side of the body or the other. In some cases complete recovery takes place in a few days or weeks. The vast majority of people have sufficient return of function to permit walking, some with a brace and some without. Unfortunately, a small group of patients do not recover enough muscle power to use their arms again.

2. Can a stroke cause loss of sensation in parts of the body?

It is always fascinating to think that millions of years ago the only forms of animal life on this planet were organisms which had no brains at all but were still able to live and reproduce. These animals lived in the sea (and still do), and though they were very primitive, they did have nervous systems, but quite different from ours.

The purpose of the nervous system, then and now, is to inform the animal of what is happening all around him and then make it possible for him to react to the information. For example, an animal's *sense organs* bring in the information that his enemy is near, and then his *movement system* gets him away from the enemy. Or, if he is hungry, the sense organs might signal the presence of food, and the animal would move toward the food in order to engulf it or eat it. In other words, the most basic and primitive functions of the nervous system are to bring information to the animal and then produce action. The production of action, or what we know as movement, was described in the preceding answer. This answer deals with bringing information to the animal; this is done through our body sensations.

What are these body sensations? We take them for granted, but they include a number of different kinds of information. If you close your eyes and a variety of things are done to your right hand, for example, you will be aware of each of them. You will recognize a pinprick or a blow with a hammer as painful; you can distinguish hot from cold; you can feel a feathery touch or hard pressure; vibrations or two pointed objects touching the skin at the same time can be felt. Perhaps of the greatest importance, there are sense organs in the joints which allow one to know the position of every body part *without looking*. All of these are called *sensory modalities*, and they send information along nerves, then into the spinal cord, and on up into the brain where the information is used for the benefit of the individual. Figure 2-2 shows a schematic idea of how sensory information is brought to the brain and how motor (movement) instructions are sent back out to the limbs. Notice that there is communication between the sensation interpretation areas of the brain and the movement center which initiates the process of movement in the arm. Also notice the very important fact that sensation on the right side of the body is interpreted in the left half of the brain and vice versa, just as movement of one side of the body is controlled by the opposite side of the brain.

With this background information let us return to the original question: Does a stroke cause loss of body sensations? The answer is that sometimes it does and sometimes it does not. When it does, however, it can now be understood why, and what the consequences are.

If you will refer to Figure 2-2 once more, you will see a shaded area in the lower part of the brain. If this is the part of the brain involved in the stroke, it can be seen that there may be interference with both the information being brought *to* the sensory area and *from* the movement area. Fortunately, both of these pathways are not always involved in a stroke, and so all patients do not have losses of sensation. In addition, certain patients lose some of the ability to feel

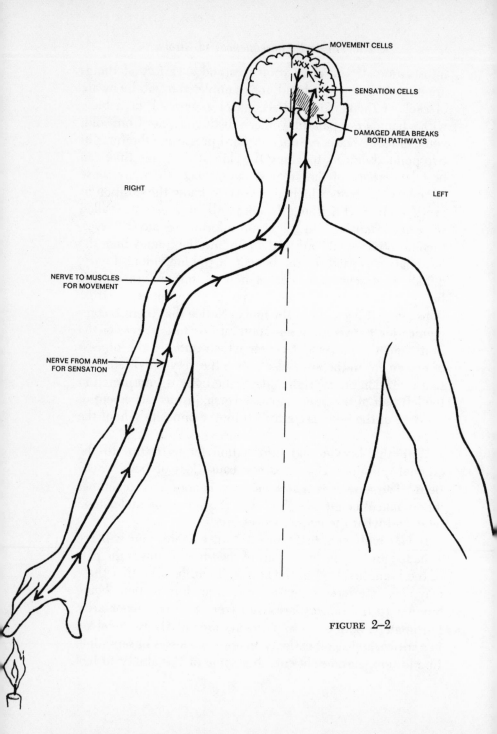

MOVEMENT CELLS

SENSATION CELLS

DAMAGED AREA BREAKS
BOTH PATHWAYS

RIGHT

LEFT

NERVE TO MUSCLES
FOR MOVEMENT

NERVE FROM ARM
FOR SENSATION

FIGURE 2–2

painful sensations but retain the sense of the position of body parts or vice versa. In other words, there may be only partial losses of sensation.

3. How may a stroke affect vision?

A stroke may affect vision in a number of ways but, fortunately, not at all in many cases. Roughly 20 percent of patients with stroke suffer some visual disturbance. The most common problem after a stroke is the partial loss of what is called the *peripheral field of vision.*

As everyone knows, the eyes are something like twin cameras. In a camera, light rays enter the small hole behind the glass lens and strike the film. This causes an image to form on the film which, after development, is the finished picture.

In the eye, the light rays enter through the pupil and strike the retina at the back of the eye. Here the similarity to a camera ends, for when these rays strike the retina they cause hundreds of thousands of cells to be activated. These cells send impulses into the brain which in turn activate other cells that are the ones which actually cause us to see (Figure 2-3 shows this process). In other words, one doesn't "see" unless this entire mechanism is working. Vision can be lost if the pupil is covered over, if the retina isn't working, or if there is damage to the optic pathway or to the cells which actually produce the picture we "see."

This is, of course, a simplification of how the visual system works, but it is sufficient for our purposes. One must know a few other facts, however, to understand how part of the field of vision may be lost.

We have pointed out that one side of the brain controls many functions on the opposite side of the body. This is true for the peripheral fields of vision which are best described as those things we see out of the corner of our eyes when we

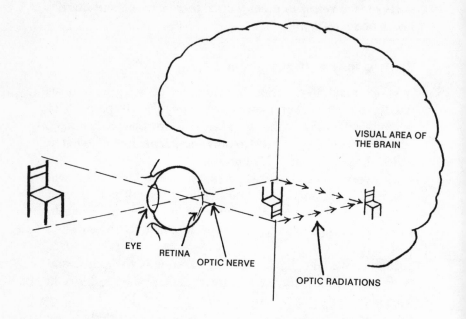

VISUAL AREA OF
THE BRAIN

EYE   RETINA
OPTIC NERVE

OPTIC RADIATIONS

FIGURE 2–3

are looking straight ahead. Direct vision is rarely affected in stroke; it is most commonly the peripheral vision which is disturbed. Thus, for example, if there is damage to the left side of the brain, the right peripheral field of vision of *both eyes* may be lost. Perhaps Figure 2-4 will clarify this.

What this loss means in practical terms is that this person will see what is directly in front of him just as well as he did before the stroke, but he will not see things "out of the corner of the eyes" to the right. This may not seem very important because we take for granted the many things which are seen in these peripheral fields. When this part of vision is lost, the patient often ignores things happening on that side because he is unaware of them. He may bump into walls on the right, ignore food on the right side of the plate, or fail to read the right side of a printed page.

It is obviously important to know whether the patient has such a problem. It may explain behavior which otherwise seems strange, and it is surprising how often one must remind the patient, particularly in the early stages, that this difficulty exists.

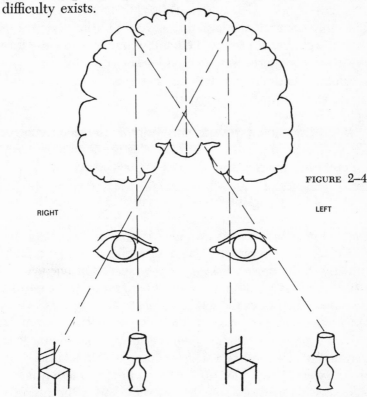

RIGHT

LEFT

FIGURE 2–4

Patients can be trained to overcome this problem by moving the head and eyes in the direction of loss. What was previously seen "out of the corner of the eyes" can then be seen by direct vision.

It should be clearly understood that this problem cannot be solved by wearing glasses, since it has nothing to do with how good the patient's vision is. A stroke doesn't affect visual acuity—that is, whether someone has 20/20 or 20/200 vision. Eyeglasses are prescribed either to magnify or make things smaller. This is not the stroke patient's problem.

Other visual problems are much less common than this. One of these is the total loss of vision in the eye on the same side as the brain damage and opposite to the hemiplegia. This only occurs if the large blood vessel in the neck (carotid) is occluded at or near the point where it branches off to the eye. This interferes with the blood supply to the eye and results in blindness, but only in that eye. In this case both direct and peripheral vision are lost since the entire eye is not functioning.

A third possible problem with vision is the occurrence of *double vision* following the stroke. This is due to an entirely different mechanism from those described. It has to do with the eyes working together.

One of the things we take for granted in vision is the fact that both eyes focus on an object and the two images, one from each retina, are seen as one. An important part of this process is the accurate movement of each eye so that it looks directly at the object. If some of the muscles of one eye are paralyzed or weak, it may not be able to move in the desired direction; therefore, the image on that retina will not be in the proper place, so to speak, and the patient will see double.

This situation is present when the stroke causes damage to certain cells in the brain which control the eye muscles. In the answers to the previous questions in this chapter, it was described how paralysis or loss of sensation is the result of some interference in the pathway from the brain to outer parts of the body such as the skin or the muscles. Although strokes tend to occur in a certain few locations in the brain, theoretically they can occur anywhere. One of the less frequent locations is in the *brain stem,* and it is in these cases that there may be double vision. It can be seen from Figure

2-5 how such a stroke could interfere with movements of the eye and result in double vision.

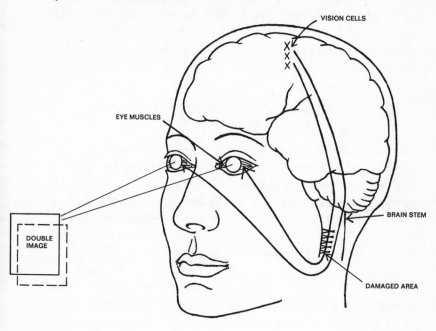

VISION CELLS

EYE MUSCLES

BRAIN STEM

DOUBLE IMAGE

DAMAGED AREA

FIGURE 2–5

Finally, the fourth type of eye difficulty, one that is seen about as frequently as double vision, is known as *nystagmus*. This is a continuous, rhythmic movement of the eyes which is involuntary and which is again due to damage in the brain stem. The eyes may move in this fashion in almost any direction, but most commonly they move in the horizontal plane. This is less disturbing to the patient than the other problems mentioned, but it is annoying because of the constant movement; it makes it more difficult to see things clearly.

It should be pointed out that strokes involving the brain

41

stem can affect both sides of the body, therefore both eyes, because the brain stem is like a passageway from the brain to the outer parts of the body, like the eyes, the mouth, the arms and legs. This can be seen in Figures 2–5 and 2–7. Therefore nystagmus affects both eyes, double vision either one or both.

4. Why do some patients have jerky movements of the arm and leg after a stroke?

In the answer to Question 1 the role of the brain in controlling body movements was described. It will be recalled that any movement is initiated by the action of certain cells in the most advanced part of the brain, the cortex. Before these impulses or firings can produce a certain movement, they must "ignite" other cells, which in turn cause muscles to contract and, therefore, movement to occur.

This seems like a rather simple process, but it is not the whole story. In order for the movements of an arm to be smooth, there must be feedback into the brain at all times. In other words while the brain is saying "Now move out and pick up that glass," the arm must be sending messages back to the brain which say "I am now 4 feet away from the glass, now 3 feet, now 2 feet, etc." as well as "The fingers are beginning to open, now they are fully open, now they are beginning to close around the glass." Unless there is a constant stream of information going back into the brain, it does not know how to regulate the movement of the arm. A loss of such regulation is seen as jerky movements and is called *ataxia* or *incoordination*.

There are two situations in stroke which may produce ataxia. If there is no feedback from an arm, for example, which informs the brain of the position of the arm (as described in Question 2 on losses of sensation), then the brain will not have sufficient information to produce a smooth movement. The second situation is that in which the stroke occurs in the brain stem.

There is a structure in the brain which has not been mentioned before and which was designed by nature to take the major responsibility for proper coordination. It is called the *cerebellum* and is located near the brain stem. All the feedback from the arms, legs, eyes—in fact all moving parts of the body—goes into the cerebellum, which in some way that is not yet fully understood by scientists sees to it that movements remain smooth. (See Figure 2–6.)

Strokes which occur in or near the brain stem may interfere with this very delicate mechanism. As a result, move-

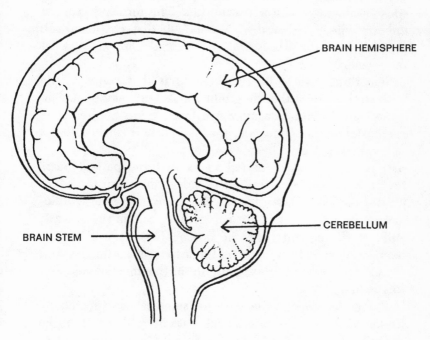

FIGURE 2–6

ments are jerky or incoordinated, and the patient may have great difficulty walking or using his arms properly.

In order to answer this question completely it should be pointed out that a person's balance may be disturbed by the same process. Someone who is drunk has a balance problem and damage to the brain stem may produce a similar difficulty.

5. Does a stroke affect hearing or smell?

There are hearing centers on both sides of the brain, and a stroke affects only one side. As pointed out in Question 15, Chapter 3, one must not confuse a problem in *understanding* spoken language with a hearing loss. The former is part of *aphasia* which is described in detail in that chapter. Such patients hear the words very well but do not know what they mean.

Something else to be remembered is that many people with strokes are in the age group where they may be having some trouble with hearing. Since hearing loss is often slow and insidious in coming on, the patient and sometimes his family may not have been aware of it.

It is occasionally reported to us that the patient hears better if spoken to on the "good" side rather than the hemiplegic side. The reason for this is not entirely clear. Audiometric testing is usually normal for both ears in such a case, and yet the patient states he doesn't hear as well on the hemiplegic side. Some doctors think there is an unconscious "extinction" of the sounds going in on the affected side, but this is theoretical.

To our knowledge the sense of smell is not affected by stroke. However, an occasional patient will say that he doesn't taste food as he did before, and since the sense of smell is part of taste there may be an involvement of this mechanism.

6. Does a stroke affect the functioning of internal organs?

There is still a great deal which is not known about the effect of a stroke on the body. For example, almost all people who have suffered strokes complain for many months after of excessive fatigue. One might expect this for two or three months as part of the convalescent period, but when it extends for months beyond there must be another explanation. Undoubtedly, research will be done to clarify this problem.

There is some evidence that the respiratory mechanism is affected after a stroke. The breathing muscles of the chest do not seem to work as well on the hemiplegic side of the body, and as a consequence the exchange of carbon dioxide for fresh oxygen which occurs in the lungs is not quite as efficient. The full consequences of this have not yet been thoroughly studied.

With regard to the heart, the kidneys, and the digestive system, we do not know of any direct effect of stroke on these.

Of course, immediately after the onset of a stroke, the patient's state of consciousness may be reduced and many of his internal functions will be altered. He may not have control of his urine, for example, but this is usually transient and does not represent a permanent change produced by the stroke.

Some patients have a change in bowel habits after a stroke, but it is not important though it may be annoying.

7. What does handedness have to do with a stroke?

One of the two halves of the brain (hemispheres) is said to be *preferred* in the great majority of human beings. This means that the arm and leg which that side of the brain controls are the ones the patient uses best—and that is what is meant by handedness. Therefore, if a stroke occurs in the left hemisphere of a person who is right-handed, it means that the preferred side of his brain has been involved, and he will lose function in the arm and leg he uses best.

8. What do you notice when you look at someone who has had a stroke?

Usually there is a droop of one side of the face, the eyelid may not be open as wide, the corner of the mouth will be down. If it is a very mild stroke, one will notice only that the nose is slightly flat on one side. The involved arm may hang loosely at the side or be bent somewhat at the elbow, wrist, and fingers. When the stroke patient is standing still, one may not suspect any trouble with the leg, but when he begins to walk it will seem as though the involved leg is heavy and hard to lift off the ground. When it does move it may look very mechanical and stiff; there may be very little bending of the knee, and the foot may be turned inward when it is off the ground.

In patients who recover quickly, all of this disappears in a matter of a few days or weeks; in others it persists for longer periods.

9. Can you describe the physical changes which occur right after a stroke and how they recover?

It is important to remember that in many cases recovery from a stroke is very rapid and physical changes may be present for just a few hours or days. These patients usually require a number of weeks for convalescence despite the fact that there is no problem with movement, sensation, or vision.

Now let us consider the sequence of events which occurs in someone who does not have a quick return of function. The onset of the stroke is, by definition, sudden. In the majority of cases there is no loss of consciousness. The arm and leg on one side become limp, the face on that side usually sags, sensation may be lost. Often patients fall or slump over because of the sudden loss of movement on one side.

During the next two to three days the affected arm and leg will remain limp; that is, the paralysis will be of the kind in which the limbs are like those of a rag doll. This is called *flaccid paralysis;* it lasts for a short time in some patients and much longer in others. The patient is not able to walk and requires complete nursing care. As soon as possible, he is encouraged to sit on the edge of the bed and then in an easy chair.

What happens to the limp arm and leg? The first step in the process of recovery is that the limbs develop more *tone;* that is, despite the patient's inability to move his arm or leg, it now has more life. If the doctor tries to move the limb very quickly it will automatically resist a little. This increase in tone is called *spasticity,* and unless recovery goes on to completion it may persist and become more severe.

The next step is the beginning of *voluntary movement,* which means the person can move the paralyzed limb on his own. Usually the leg recovers before the arm, and it is the thigh segment of the leg which first moves. At about this same time one may observe that whenever the patient flexes his thigh, the knee also bends and the ankle bends upward. The knee and ankle movements are automatic or *reflex movements,* as they are properly called, and are part of the recovery process. In the meantime, spasticity has been getting worse.

The final step, if recovery of movement is destined to go on to completion, is that the person begins to move all parts of the limb independently of each other and with greater

47

and greater strength. At the same time that this is occurring, spasticity diminishes in intensity, and when there is complete control of the limb again, the spasticity is gone.

What all of this means is that the cortex of the brain is once more in normal contact with the limbs. It is the highest control center in the brain, and when it has been partially or completely cut off from the limbs, as occurs in a stroke, paralysis and spasticity are the result.

Sagging of one side of the face, which is really the same as paralysis of the arm and leg, gradually improves. The patient is usually left only with a mild asymmetry of the face after a few months, if he does not recover completely.

The recovery of normal sensation is not as complicated as that of movement. In a sense, it either does or it doesn't return. If sufficient healing occurs in the involved area of the brain, the person usually recovers sensation in a few weeks. If there is still a problem after three months, it may be permanent.

10. Can a person have involvement of both sides of the body after a stroke?

In the great majority of strokes the symptoms are on one side of the body only. Occasionally, the damaged area is in the *brain stem* and may affect both sides. Figure 2-7 illustrates why this is so.

The shaded area (damaged part) involves pathways to both the right arm and left arm, and there may be trouble in both. Fortunately, this is quite rare.

11. How does the doctor decide how much damage the stroke did?

In most cases, it does not require a doctor to know that someone has had a stroke, but as the preceding answers have

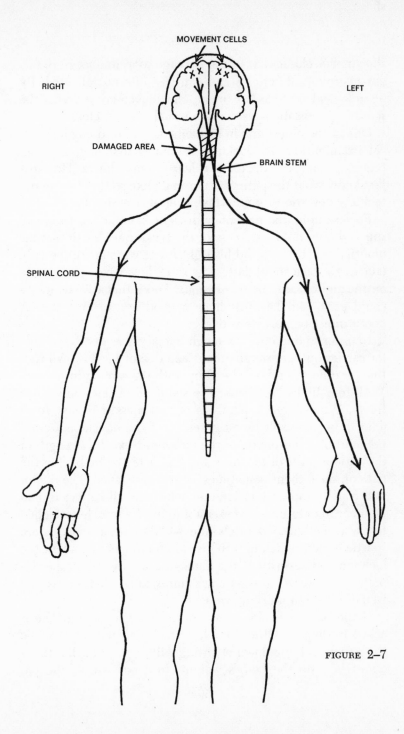

MOVEMENT CELLS

RIGHT

LEFT

DAMAGED AREA

BRAIN STEM

SPINAL CORD

FIGURE 2–7

shown, a stroke may result in damage to a number of different neurological systems and can be quite complicated. By neurological systems we mean the movement system, the sensory or sensation system, the visual system, etc.

One of the oldest arts in medicine is that of doing a physical examination. By looking, listening, touching, moving, pinching, etc., the doctor can learn many things. He must first know what the patient is normally like so that he can detect any deviation from normal, even if it is slight.

For example, the patient with right hemiplegia may have suffered only mild weakness of the facial muscles so that his mouth doesn't droop and his right eye is wide open; the only clue might be a slight flattening of the lower part of the nose on the right side. The doctor must know that this symptom could exist, and he must have a good eye to detect it. A doctor must be part detective.

In order to find out how much damage was done, the doctor carries out an examination. Each doctor has his own routine for doing this, but all end up with the same information.

All four limbs are checked to see if all of the joints move freely. When there is paralysis or weakness it is easy for a joint to become stiff by a tightening of the envelope around the joint or a shortening of the muscles. Next the strength of the various parts of the arms and legs is tested by having the patient move them, sometimes against resistance. The doctor will usually tap certain tendons with a small rubber-tipped hammer to determine the excitability of the muscles attached to these tendons. This tells him whether these muscles are spastic or not, which in turn gives him information about the location and severity of the damage done by the stroke. Finally, he observes the patient's limbs to see if there is any tremor or involuntary movement.

If the patient is able to stand and take some steps, he is asked to do this. Often muscles which will not move while the patient is lying down or sitting will respond to the stimulus of bearing the body's weight. In other words, the patient's leg does not crumple when he stands on it—which means that the muscles must be contracting. If asked to move the leg (contract the muscles) while lying down, the patient may not be able to do so. This is obviously important since it is essential that the patient walk if he can possibly do so.

Next, the doctor may examine the sensory system. He checks to see if the patient can feel a simple touch, then pricks the skin with a pin to determine if he still feels pain normally. He may then touch the skin with a vibrating tuning fork to see if this type of sensation is perceived normally, and, finally, the doctor may move the patient's fingers or toes (with the patient's eyes closed) to see if he can tell in which direction they were moved. This last test is particularly important since, as described before, the sense of position or knowing automatically where the body parts are is essential to normal movement. When this sense is lost the patient must *look* in order to see where the limbs are, and his movements become jerky and uncoordinated.

The doctor may then move on to examine the patient's head. He first notes if the facial muscles are weak, whether the lips move properly, whether the tongue is weak or uncoordinated, whether the muscles of the throat are working properly, whether sensation in the mouth and throat is normal. He then may check the eyes to see if they move well in all directions (if they don't, the person may have double vision) and whether there is involuntary movement. He tests for visual ability when the patient is looking straight ahead and then checks the peripheral fields (see Question 3 for a complete discussion of this). The doctor tests peripheral vision by asking the patient to look straight ahead and wiggling a finger off to the side. If the peripheral fields are lost, the patient will not be able to see the finger "out of the corner of his eye."

While he is conducting this examination, the doctor is observing how much the patient can speak and understand, how well he follows instructions, and a host of other things

51

which tell him about the extent of damage which may have been done.

It is the nervous system which is primarily involved in a stroke, although the trouble starts in a blood vessel. By nervous system we mean the brain and the intricate connections between the brain and the rest of the body. If there is damage to the brain, it results in malfunction of different parts of the body. In doing the physical examination and noting what has changed in the functioning of the body, the doctor, through his knowledge of anatomy, has an idea of what part of the brain was damaged and how severely. There are other means of getting such information. The next question deals with these.

12. What tests are done after someone has had a stroke?

Tests are done to give the doctor more information than he can obtain from a physical examination. Why is this information important? Because although most strokes look alike, they are not all caused by the same thing. This has been discussed in some detail in Chapter 1.

It is *always* important to know exactly what caused a stroke in order to know whether anything can or should be done to treat it. The best example of what we mean is the stroke caused by a brain tumor. Although these are not common, they are often treatable by surgical removal of the tumor with subsequent clearing of the stroke. But the doctor must know that it is a tumor and not a thrombosis which has caused the stroke.

Similarly, ruptured blood vessels can often be surgically treated and the hemorrhage evacuated if one knows that a hemorrhage is the cause of the stroke.

Probably the most commonly done test is an examination of the spinal fluid. A sample of this fluid is safely and simply obtained by inserting a thin needle low down in the spinal canal. By sight or by laboratory examination it can be determined if there is blood in the fluid (there should not be); other tests show whether it has the right quantities of various substances which are normally found in spinal fluid.

Plain X-rays of the skull are also part of the routine for just about every patient. When read by a skilled radiologist or neurologist, a great deal of information can be gained about certain structures in the brain, as well as the skull itself. For more detailed information other types of X-rays are done which yield much more information; these will be described below.

The electroencephalograph (EEG) or "brain-wave machine" is well known to most people and provides another test which is simple to do and sometimes very helpful. Wired metal tabs or tiny needles are attached to the skull and the electrical waves which the brain makes by its normal activity are transmitted through the wires to a machine where they make a record of wavy lines. The shape of these lines may be read by an expert as normal or as indicating trouble somewhere in the brain. The EEG cannot distinguish between a thrombosis or a hemorrhage, but it is sometimes very helpful to the neurologist by pointing the finger of suspicion at one part of the brain or another.

A test which has come into use recently employs a safe radioactive substance which is injected into the blood stream. As it goes through the circulatory system it goes through the brain, sending off rays of radioactivity as it goes. An X-ray film is placed near the skull, and as the rays emerge from the brain they cause changes on the X-ray film very much as light rays produce a photograph in a camera. Abnormalities within the substance of brain tissue sometimes show up in these special "radiographs." This technique goes by the general name of *radioactive scanning*.

If the neurologist does not obtain all the information he

needs from the foregoing tests, there are two others which are available, and sometimes these are the only ones which give enough information. They are the *pneumoencephalogram* and the *arteriogram*.

In the first test, a quantity of air is injected into the empty spaces (empty except for cerebrospinal fluid) located in the center of the brain. Air shows up on X-ray film as dark shadows compared to the surrounding tissue, and as a consequence the spaces are outlined. Now if something is pressing into one of the spaces, it will show up on the X-ray since the shape of the space will be abnormal. Figure 2–8 illustrates this.

Although relatively new compared to the other tests described, the arteriogram is perhaps the most valuable of all because it outlines the blood vessels of the brain. A harmless substance is injected into the blood vessel system and travels all over the body. As it passes through the brain, twelve X-rays are taken very rapidly, and the blood vessels show up very clearly on the X-ray film. These reveal whether the blood vessels are open, whether they are narrow or sometimes too wide, whether there is a weak spot on a vessel, whether something is pressing on an artery or vein, or whether one of them is in the wrong position. It is a very valuable test, and when done by experienced, trained people it is completely safe.

In addition to these special tests there are a number of blood tests which are sometimes helpful in learning the cause of a stroke. Everyone is familiar with how blood samples are secured.

When the history of the illness, the physical examination, and the tests are all taken together, the physician is as close to knowing the cause of a stroke as he can be.

The time to concentrate on finding the cause for stroke and therefore the time to do these tests is immediately after it has happened. It bears repeating that the neurologist will decide which ones should be done; sometimes very few are indicated.

Some of these tests are done before a stroke if someone is having symptoms which suggest the possibility that a stroke will occur. Many people have avoided a stroke through prompt testing and the application of proper treatment.

13. What is spasticity?

This is a question which is only asked by an occasional patient who is receiving rehabilitation therapy or by a member of his family. The doctor or a therapist may use the word in response to someone's question about why the hemiplegic arm or leg reacts as it does.

The full explanation of spasticity is too complicated to attempt here, but it can be described. It refers to a stiffness or tightness in the patient's muscles and is present only when the muscles are weak; as they regain their power, the spasticity disappears.

There are a number of ways to tell if a muscle is spastic. If the patient's arm is suddenly moved by the examiner it will automatically resist. For instance, if the elbow is slowly bent and then suddenly straightened out, it will resist. Another way is to tap the tendon of a spastic muscle, as is often done at the knee. If there is spasticity the leg will jump more than it normally should.

Sometimes one can suspect the presence of spasticity simply by looking at the patient. If the hand tends to curl up and the wrist remains bent, it is likely that the muscles which cause these positions are spastic.

Question 13 in Chapter 5 discusses the treatment for spasticity. The most important thing to remember is that spasticity will gradually disappear as muscles regain normal strength.

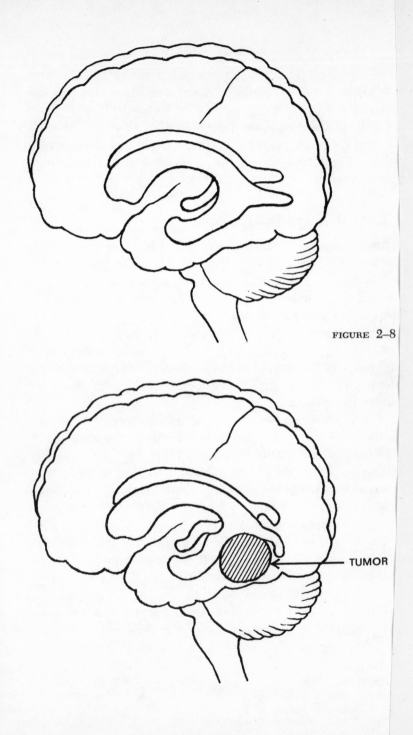

FIGURE 2–8

TUMOR

14. Why does the patient's paralyzed arm move when he yawns? Does it mean the arm is getting better?

Many of the body's movements are automatic; the medical term for this is reflex. It means that the higher centers of the brain do not have to participate in bringing about such movements. They will occur automatically if something triggers them.

For example, if a cinder flies into an eye, the eyelids automatically blink. This eye-blink does not require the participation of cortical cells. Similarly, if one's hand touches a lighted cigarette, the arm will pull back very quickly—again, a reflex. There are a great variety of things which can set off reflexes. The pressure of one's foot on the ground stimulates a reflex that causes the leg to straighten out so that the body's weight can be borne. Most reflexes are independent of the higher centers of the brain although they may be modified by them. Therefore, if these centers are damaged by a stroke so that some part of the body, like the right arm, cannot be moved voluntarily, that arm may be able to move automatically since the higher centers are not part of the reflex mechanism.

Stretching the arms with a yawn is a reflex, and one may be astonished to see the paralyzed arm move when the patient yawns. Unfortunately, it cannot be interpreted to mean that function is returning to the arm, since it is a reflex and has nothing to do with the damaged area of the brain.

Incidentally, the same type of thing is at work when a patient's arm or fingers move at night while he is asleep.

15. Why does the patient's arm stiffen when he walks?

This is related to what happens when he yawns, which was discussed in the preceding answer.

There are connections between all parts of the body, and very often what happens in one part may cause things to happen in other parts. For example, when a person walks his arms swing. This is automatic or, to use the medical term, it is a reflex. When the right leg moves forward so does the left arm and vice versa.

After a stroke these connections are still intact in the spinal cord, but they no longer work properly as far as the hemiplegic side is concerned. The movement of the legs in walking stimulates the hemiplegic arm to move, but not normally. Instead it is drawn up into a bent position.

16. Why is it that sometimes a person's leg will get better but not his arm?

Perhaps Figure 2–9 can illustrate this best.

There are cells in the brain which are responsible for each part of the body. Messages or impulses go out from these cells to the parts of the body for which they are responsible —these pathways are shown in Figure 2–9. Now if the area of damage from the stroke is in the way of these message pathways, it can be seen that there will be interference with movement. The shaded area is the damaged part of the brain. In this case more of the arm pathways are involved than the leg. Therefore, it is easy to see how the leg would recover function while the arm might not.

In the same way one often sees a patient whose upper arm can move but who has no motion in the wrist and fingers. The message pathways to the upper arm have been spared but those to the hand must lie within the damaged zone. The messages are not transmitted and the hand cannot move.

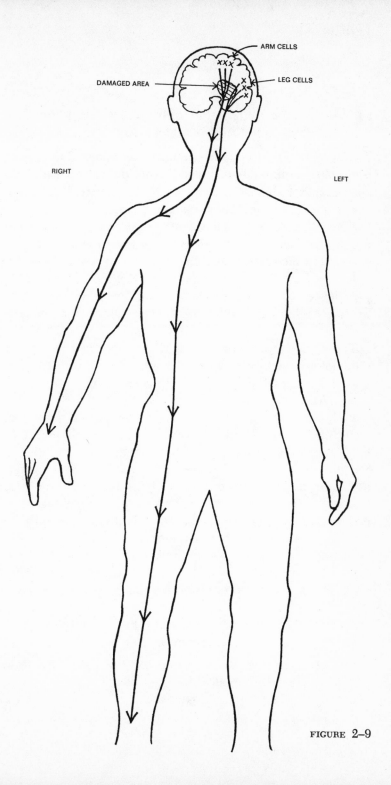

ARM CELLS

DAMAGED AREA

LEG CELLS

RIGHT

LEFT

FIGURE 2–9

17. Why is the patient not able to use his hand very well even though he has good strength in it?

This may be due to one of a number of things. The loss of *position sense* in the hand makes it very difficult to use it in a coordinated fashion. To understand this better, reread the answers to Questions 2 and 4 in this chapter.

It will be recalled that smooth, coordinated movements require feedback from the limb being used—the hand in this case. If the feedback is lost, the patient will encounter great difficulty. In his book *Episode,** Eric Hodgins describes his experiences related to the loss of position sense. They are worth reading for both their neurological and literary qualities.

The second possible reason is that the patient may have something called *apraxia* of the hand. This is an extremely difficult concept to explain, mainly because we do not fully comprehend what causes it ourselves. We know that it is frequently seen in a patient who has had a stroke and that it has something to do with the chain of command in the brain. It is as though the hand has the normal ability to move, that is, the muscles are working properly, but the brain is not capable of issuing the correct orders to the hand. Fortunately, this seems to improve after a few months, but while it is present, it is very perplexing to the patient and his family. It is very important that family members try to find out from the doctor if the patient has apraxia so that they will know that he is not being stubborn about not using his hand. The same is true for any other problem that is not fully understood.

Finally, the patient may not use his hand because he *doesn't know it's there.* This is even more difficult to believe,

* Eric Hodgins, *Episode: Report on the Accident in My Skull,* Atheneum Publishers, New York, 1964, pp. 202–204.

but it is often seen during the period immediately after a stroke. It is as though the patient has forgotten that he has an arm and leg on the involved side. We sometimes say that he "denies" the existence of these limbs, but it is probably more accurate to say that he is not aware of their presence. This, too, recovers fairly promptly since it is rare to find it in a patient two to three months after a stroke.

It must be repeated whenever one sees any strange, unexplainable behavior, it is wise to consult a physician and find out its cause. We have seen family members worry unnecessarily or, worse, berate the patient about his inability to use his hand when the reason for it was quite obvious. Knowledge dispels worry and fear; it helps us avoid mistakes; it helps build constructive attitudes about the patient's physical problems and what can be done about them.

18. Why is the patient's balance poor when he first begins to walk?

This may be attributed to a number of things, not all of which are present in each patient.

One of the commonest reasons is the weakness of the hemiplegic leg. The patient attempts to put his weight on the leg, and since it can't hold him very well, he tends to fall over. In time the leg regains strength, and this is no longer a problem.

In some cases it is really a question of balance. Some part of the equilibrium mechanism of the brain is damaged, and the patient tends to fall.

Other patients have this trouble because they do not see things as they are. For example, the room may appear tilted, depth perception may be disturbed, objects distorted, or foreground and background mixed up.

Another common reason is the absence of position sense in the foot and leg. If the brain does not have feedback on the position of the leg, it cannot give accurate orders about where to put it. This makes for incoordination and poor balance.

All of these problems can be overcome, since the great majority of patients learn to walk no matter how severe the stroke.

19. Why is the patient afraid of falling?

The answer to the preceding question could also be the answer to this one. The patient's fear of falling is natural in view of all the problems he has to cope with in walking. This fear is almost always overcome.

20. Why is the patient so tired?

We touched on this problem in Question 6. It probably affects the great majority of stroke patients and, to our knowledge, the reason for it is unknown. It is expected that the patient will fatigue easily during the first few months; this is the period of convalescence. But it is quite common for this to continue for as long as eighteen or twenty-four months and, in some cases, even longer.

One might as well be aware of this since it must be considered in planning for the future. It means that even though a man can return to his old job, it is best to plan on reducing the hours or intensity of work. A housewife ought not count on doing as much as she did prior to the illness.

One can speculate on the cause of persistent fatigue even though we have no evidence for any of these speculations. Since the brain is so important to all body functions, it is entirely possible that the stroke interferes with some glandular or metabolic function. Why this goes on so long is a mystery.

A second possibility is that the patient's natural depression (which will be discussed in greater detail in Chapter 4) is the cause of this lack of energy. Depression can make someone feel completely washed out, and since every patient is depressed for quite a while after a stroke, this could be the cause. Against this is the fact that the patient usually recovers his energy after resting; one would expect that a rest would make little difference to a depressed person. They tend to be lethargic all the time.

In Question 6 we suggested the possibility that a mild impairment of respiratory function may be the cause.

Perhaps it is foolish to speculate at length since there are so many possibilities. This is a mystery which can only be solved by systematic research. One can be confident, however, that the solution will eventually be found.

21. Should the patient have extra rest every day?

In view of the previous question on fatigue it is clear that most patients need extra rest during the day. How much will depend upon the individual situation. It is natural and necessary under the circumstances.

22. Does a patient's sleep pattern change after a stroke?

Sleeping habits do change in the great majority of patients. Almost universally, the family will tell you that the patient sleeps well and long—even if he didn't before. Perhaps this is related to the easy fatigability mentioned in Question 20. Sleeping long hours is *not* a bad sign and does not imply that the patient is not doing well.

Less commonly, a person may not sleep as much after a stroke. The most likely explanation for this is anxiety, which is certainly understandable under the circumstances.

23. Why does the stroke patient stop smoking?

Not all do. In those who do it is usually a reflection of the change in personality which may occur for a while after the stroke. The patient may drop many of his old habits, sometimes permanently.

Another way of looking at this is that patients frequently lose their anxiety after a stroke. We see this, and it has been described by people who have had strokes. Patients will often say they don't worry about their families, don't worry about finances, have no concern for the future. Since smoking is usually a way of working off nervous tension and since the stroke may eliminate tension, the patient stops smoking.

24. Do the patient's tastes in food and drink change?

Frequently they do and this is related to dropping the smoking habit, since eating, like smoking, is a common means of working off tension.

However, in some patients there is a total disinterest in eating which may be a result of depression or merely another change in habit.

We do not really understand this very well, but it is no cause for concern. Most Americans eat too much anyway, and we have never seen a patient who suffered because of his eating habits.

Occasionally real problems, like alcoholism, disappear completely. We recall a lady who had been an alcoholic for years and never touched a drop after her stroke. This is not the recommended cure for alcohol addiction, but it shows that the results of a stroke are not all tragic.

25. What does pain in the hemiplegic arm mean?

In most patients pain in the arm is related to disuse. That is, because of weakness or paralysis the arm is not moved; it hangs heavily and stretches ligaments, at the shoulder particularly, which produces pain. It has been our experience with many different kinds of conditions that a body part which does not move normally tends to become painful. The muscles themselves become painful. The proof of this is that the pain usually disappears as function returns. Even if the arm does not become normal, the increased activity tends to reduce the pain.

Another cause of pain is something called the *shoulder–band syndrome*. Its medical name is *reflex sympathetic dystrophy,* and it is characterized by pain in the entire arm, but most severely in the shoulder and hand, swelling of a particular type in the hand, coldness of the hand, and X-ray findings in the bones of the hand and wrist which are quite typical. It is believed to be caused by excessive discharge of the sympathetic nervous system into the hemiplegic arm, but why that occurs is still a mystery.

Your doctor has a method of treatment for this. It is interesting that one group of doctors has found that intensive physical therapy with treatments a few times a day is very effective. This leads one to think that this problem, too, may be related to disuse of the hemiplegic arm.

Another cause of pain in the hemiplegic arm is the result of damage to an area of the brain which has to do with transmitting feelings to the sensation interpretation portion of the brain. It is a kind of way station called the *thalamus,* and occasionally a patient will experience pain in an arm or leg because the thalamus has been injured. Fortunately, this type of pain is rare, since it may be very difficult to control.

Various segments of the arm may be painful because the joints have been allowed to get stiff or tight. This is becoming inexcusable since it is common knowledge now that the hemiplegic limbs must be exercised and kept limber even if they are totally paralyzed.

Whatever the reason for pain, there are usually ways of relieving it. Your doctor will know what to do. Except in these specific instances, pain is not part of the stroke syndrome.

26. Why do some patients have trouble controlling bladder and bowel function after a stroke?

If this occurs it is temporary in the great majority of patients. It happens because the brain is involved in all body functions in one way or another. A stroke often results in temporary malfunctioning because of swelling in brain tissues. In time this *edema fluid* is absorbed, and the disturbed body function returns to normal.

One of the parts of the brain that may be so affected after a stroke has to do with awareness. In essence the patient becomes confused. This confusion may extend to some of the bodily functions, like controlling the bladder, and result in failure to control urine. (The subject of confusion is taken up in greater detail in Chapter 4).

To repeat, it is only temporary in most patients, and one should not conclude that it is a bad sign.

27. What happens to the blood pressure after a stroke?

Nature is often kind while she is being most harsh, and so it is with the blood pressure after a stroke. It usually falls to normal or near normal levels. This is one of those phenomena for which we have no good explanation, but undoubtedly as we learn more about stroke the reason will become apparent.

28. What is a seizure?

As with so many things pertaining to illness, there is a mystery and fear associated with seizure that is unwarranted. Nothing about illness is pleasant, but many conditions are feared beyond reason. Perhaps it is because fear itself is beyond reason.

A seizure is a sudden firing off of a large number of brain cells at the same time producing contraction of many different muscles. This is why one or more parts of the body may become stiff during a seizure. It is sometimes, but not always, accompanied by brief fainting. Seizures usually last only a few minutes, and the patient often sleeps after it is over. Sometimes only one limb or part of a limb will be involved.

No one really knows why seizures occur or how they actually get started, but it is known that abnormal places in the brain trigger them. For example, if there is a "scar" somewhere in the brain as a result of an old injury, it may be the place where a seizure begins. The electroencephalograph can often detect such spots in the brain.

In the majority of cases seizures can be *prevented* by the use of appropriate medications. There are now a great many of these available so that doctors can choose the best combination for the individual patient.

29. Do seizures have anything to do with stroke?

Occasionally a stroke comes on with a seizure, but it does not mean that the stroke is a severe one if this happens. Nor does it mean that the area of brain involved is large.

A small percentage of patients will have a seizure sometime after the stroke but, as stated in the last answer, these can be prevented thereafter by the use of medicines. Sometimes the doctor will administer these medications from the beginning if he suspects that a seizure might occur.

It is important to know that seizures do not cause death, and that they do not mean the patient is getting worse or will have another stroke. They do not cause bodily harm and do not increase the weakness, loss of sensation, vision problems, or any other part of the stroke.

Another myth about seizures concerns what one does if a seizure occurs. In most cases the patient has some indication that one is about to occur, and he can lie down or sit down. The best thing for those with the patient to do is nothing, except make him comfortable. It will run its course in a few minutes. A seizure is no reason for panic or alarm. When it is over the doctor should be consulted so that he can make recommendations as to treatment.

30. Does a stroke affect the wearing of dentures?

This may seem like a strange question to some, but it is very important to the person who wears dentures.

The great majority of patients will have some sagging of the face on one side after a stroke. This means that there is weakness of the facial muscles on that side. When the patient smiles the normal side will pull harder than the hemiplegic side, and the smile will be crooked. This not only affects the patient's appearance, but his speech may be somewhat slurred and his dentures may not fit as well. Actually, other changes in the mouth caused by the stroke contribute to a change in the gums and the way the tongue functions. Altogether they pose a problem for the wearer of dentures.

The best solution is for the patient not to leave his dentures out for long periods. We know this by experience. Patients who have removed their dentures and left them out usually require a new set. Those who have left them in seem to do quite well.

As we have said elsewhere, the facial sagging will improve as time goes by so that most patients will eventually show very little evidence of the original weakness.

31. Why does the patient's voice sometimes change in pitch after a stroke?

When this occurs it is usually a very slight change and often only the patient is aware of the difference. If there is any change, the voice is slightly higher in pitch. We believe this is due to the fact that the stream of air passing between vocal cords is not quite as strong as it was prior to the stroke. This tends to make the voice a trifle "tighter," which raises the pitch. Some patients complain that their voices are weaker, no doubt for the same reason.

~~~~~~

CHAPTER 3

The Speech Disorders Associated with Stroke

1. What are the different kinds of speech disorders associated with a stroke?
2. What are the symptoms of aphasia and verbal apraxia?
3. Who can have speech disorders?
4. Do speech disorders differ in severity?
5. Why can an aphasic patient say words on certain occasions and not at other times?
6. If an aphasic patient can sing and count why can't he speak?
7. Is it natural for an aphasic patient to use his native language more easily than a second language?
8. Can aphasia be temporary?
9. Can a patient sometimes read and write and yet not speak?
10. Does a patient's speech disorder ever become worse?
11. Does the patient's difficulty in reading have anything to do with vision?
12. What is the connection between eating and speech?
13. I know that the patient can say a lot of things. Why doesn't he?

14. Does the patient mean it when he swears?
15. Does a stroke cause a hearing loss?
16. Do patients understand more when the subject is familiar to them?
17. Why is it difficult for an aphasic patient to follow conversation in a crowd?
18. Is there any medicine which can cure aphasia?
19. Can hypnosis cure aphasia?
20. Will massage or physical therapy of the vocal area help aphasia?
21. What can be done to help the aphasic patient improve his language function?
22. How soon after the onset of aphasia should speech therapy begin?
23. What is a speech therapist? A speech pathologist?
24. What does the speech pathologist actually do?
25. What can a family do for an aphasic patient if a qualified speech pathologist is not available?
26. How long will the patient need speech therapy?
27. How long should speech therapy sessions be?
28. Should the patient be forced to attend speech therapy?
29. Should a family member attend speech therapy sessions with the patient?
30. Is there group speech therapy?
31. Why not teach the aphasic patient a substitute language?
32. What kinds of words do aphasic patients recover first?
33. What specific words does the therapist concentrate on at the beginning of speech therapy?
34. Should a patient with aphasia be taught how to make vowel and consonant sounds?
35. When do you start to work on reading and writing?
36. Why does the speech therapist train the patient to write with his left hand?

37. Should the patient be taught to print or to write words?
38. The speech therapist seems to use childish methods. Is this necessary?
39. Does the patient know he has aphasia?
40. Should a patient be told that he has aphasia?
41. Do aphasic patients sometimes look at newspapers even though they have a reading impairment?
42. Do aphasic patients have difficulty concentrating when reading?
43. Does a patient with aphasia have a shortened attention span?
44. Does aphasia have anything to do with mental illness?
45. How can I tell how much the patient really knows or thinks?
46. Is a patient with aphasia capable of knowing what time it is?
47. Should a patient with a speech disorder be discouraged from associating with other patients with speech problems?
48. Is it possible for a patient to become too dependent on the use of gestures?
49. How long should you wait for an aphasic patient to answer a question?
50. How should one talk to a person who has aphasia?
51. Should I let the patient know that I don't understand him?
52. Why does the patient say "yes" to some questions when it's obvious he doesn't understand them?
53. The patient talks all the time; a lot of it I can't understand. What is this?
54. Can you give me some good ideas on how I can understand someone who has very little speech?
55. Should I correct the patient?

56. Does it help to speak to the patient on his unaffected side?

57. Should a person with aphasia be encouraged or discouraged to use the telephone?

58. Why doesn't the patient read or play cards anymore when he used to enjoy these activities?

59. Will the patient's aphasia improve as his physical condition improves?

60. I heard of someone who woke up speaking normally a year after his stroke. Is this possible?

61. Is it possible for an aphasic patient to recover more language two or three years after the onset of the stroke?

62. Will a patient improve after he stops speech therapy?

63. Does the patient's speech become normal again?

64. Will the aphasic patient be able to return to his previous job?

65. What progress has been made in treating aphasia and is there research going on?

Introduction

This chapter is an elaboration of the booklet *Understanding Aphasia,* written by Martha Taylor Sarno in 1958. That work has gone through five printings and seven translations and has been read by thousands of people since its publication.

The speech disorders following stroke are perhaps the greatest cause for heartache and concern of all of the sequelae of stroke. Man is a verbal animal, and he treasures his ability to communicate above all else. Adjustment to a speech disturbance is, therefore, particularly trying.

It is hoped that this chapter will help those patients and their families who are in the midst of that difficult adjustment and that the knowledge of what these disorders are and how they have been conquered by other people will assist in the arduous process of recovery. It is equally important that all professionals who work with stroke patients understand these problems in depth.

1. What are the different kinds of speech disorders associated with a stroke?

It is important to understand very clearly exactly what the various speech problems are, how they differ from each other, and how they differ from patient to patient. Throughout this chapter we shall use the terms *speech, communication,* and *language* interchangeably, since they all refer to the ways in which people give and receive information. Basically there are three major types of speech disorders: *aphasia, verbal apraxia,* and *dysarthria.* None of these is due to a loss of intelligence.

The one which occurs most frequently in stroke is aphasia. Though the word aphasia means "loss of the power of speech," it is generally used to refer to loss of part or all of the ability to speak, gesture, understand the spoken word, read, write, or calculate. In most patients the losses are partial, and they may involve one or more of these functions.

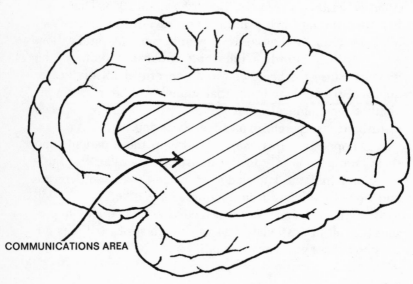

COMMUNICATIONS AREA

FIGURE 3–1

Although the ability to calculate doesn't seem to have anything to do with communication, it must be included in this group, for patients with aphasia often have simultaneous impairments in doing arithmetic.

Aphasia is most often associated with a stroke which involves the right side of the body because a part of the left side of the brain has been damaged and the centers for the control of communication are on that side. Figure 3–1 is not anatomically accurate, but it serves to illustrate the idea.

You will note that three of these language functions have to do with sending information. They are speaking, gesturing, and writing. Two of them have to do with receiving information. These are reading and understanding the spoken word. When we examine a patient to determine what type of aphasia he has, we describe it in terms of whether his problem is in sending (expression) or receiving (reception). Figure 3–2 illustrates this.

We say that a person has *expressive aphasia* if his difficulties are making his thoughts or wants known to others either through gestures, speaking, or writing. He has *receptive aphasia* if his primary difficulty is understanding what others say or understanding what he reads. Most patients with aphasia have trouble in both expression and reception; this we call *mixed aphasia*. Usually, the patient is more severely involved in one or another of these areas. The symptoms of aphasia are described in the answer to the next question.

A condition which sometimes occurs with aphasia is *verbal apraxia*. In this case the person has difficulty making the sounds of speech even though his lips, tongue, and the other muscles of speech are functioning normally. We think the trouble is to be found in a part of the brain which organizes these sounds so that they will come out as clear words, phrases, and sentences. The symptoms of verbal apraxia can be found in the answer to the next question.

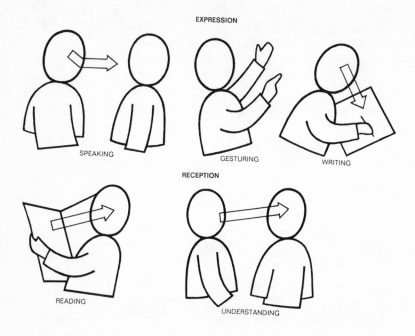

EXPRESSION

SPEAKING

GESTURING

WRITING

RECEPTION

READING

UNDERSTANDING

FIGURE 3–2

The third type of speech disorder is known as *dysarthria*. Like verbal apraxia this is a problem in which the sounds of speech are impaired, but the reason is totally different. Here one or more of the muscles of speech are impaired because of damage to a different area of the brain. This is more like the weakness which may be seen in the arm or leg when a patient has a stroke. The result is that speech sounds slurred, muddy, sometimes too loud or too soft, sometimes too slow; often the normal melody or rhythm of speech is lost. Occasionally, the quality of the voice is changed and the patient sounds as though he's talking through his nose. As we said before, this type is much less frequent after a stroke.

2. What are the symptoms of aphasia and verbal apraxia?

The most common symptoms of expressive aphasia are:

Loss of vocabulary: The patient has not really lost words. He knows what he wants to say but is prevented by his aphasia from doing so. These words are most often small ones like *by, and, or, before, the,* but any type of word can be lost. Some lose only nouns and others lose all types of words.

Word substitutions: You may hear the patient say *table* for *chair, dog* for *cat,* etc.

Perseveration: This is the repetition of a word, or sometimes just a sound, over and over. It is quite common in patients with severe aphasia, and sometimes the patient will change the word or the sound that he repeats. Severely involved patients may use only a single word repeatedly.

Jargon: This refers to what you hear when a patient has lost the ability to make real words. Instead, he puts sounds together which come out something like double-talk or a foreign language. You may think he is saying words, but when you listen closely you will realize that he is not. Obviously the patient has no control over this. Some patients know they're doing it, others don't.

Use of opposites: It is common for an aphasic to use the opposite word to the one intended. For example, *yes* for *no, he* for *she, up* for *down, in* for *out, big* for *little,* etc. He is usually not aware of this.

Circumlocution: This word is from the Latin and means literally to "speak around." When a patient has lost nouns, as some do, trying to express a thought may be very difficult. For example, instead of saying "I went to buy a pen," he might say "I went to get one of those things you use when you write a—you know, one of those things for mailing." The patient couldn't find the word "pen," and in an attempt to describe one got himself into a situation in which he had to use the word "letter," but not being able to use the word "letter" he went even farther afield. This is circumlocution.

Writing aphasia is much like speaking aphasia in that the patient may have loss of vocabulary, word substitutions, perseveration, and circumlocution. One can see all degrees of severity. Some patients can only write their names; others make very few errors. Occasionally a patient can copy words but can't write spontaneously. In a severe case, the patient may write letters which are recognizable but out of order. The result might be *teh gril slimed* instead of *the girl smiled*. Some make totally unrecognizable symbols.

Since *gestures* are a part of communication they may be lost or incorrectly used. Someone may nod "yes" for "no" or make a gesture which seems to have no meaning. This is important to understand since one often sees family members desperately trying to interpret gestures which are meaningless.

The symptoms of expressive aphasia are much more noticeable than those of *receptive aphasia*. In the latter, the most important is impaired *auditory comprehension,* which means difficulty understanding the spoken word. If the patient has only a mild problem of this kind you may not be aware of it.

A *reading deficit* may be equally confusing since it is frequently not the ability to read which is lost, but the understanding of what has been read. This is analogous to losses in understanding the spoken word. The person hears the words which are spoken, just as he reads them from the printed page, but he doesn't know what they mean. It is much like hearing or reading a foreign language.

Verbal apraxia, referred to in Question 1, sometimes accompanies aphasia. In addition to having many of the symptoms just described, the patient has trouble pronouncing the words he can say. It seems as though he can't control his tongue and makes great efforts to do so. His speech is slow and labored. Patients with verbal apraxia often have difficulty imitating speech movements. The remaining questions in this chapter will refer to aphasia unless verbal apraxia or dysarthria are specified.

As stated in Question 1, none of these symptoms reflects a loss of intelligence. They are disturbances in the communication system and can exist in the presence of normal intelligence.

3. Who can have speech disorders?

Somewhat less than half of all those who have strokes suffer a speech disorder, and there is no way to predict in which cases this will occur; age, sex, education, vocation, race, or nationality are not determining factors. Though more men have strokes than women, the same proportion of either sex will have a language disorder.

4. Do speech disorders differ in severity?

Yes. As described in Question 1 they differ in both type and severity. The most severe type, referred to as *global aphasia,* is characterized by deficits in all of the communication areas. Fortunately, many are so mild that it is impossible to detect the aphasia except in situations which require complicated speech or understanding. In some aphasic patients different elements of the aphasia vary in degree of severity. A patient, for example, may have a severe expressive aphasia accompanied by a mild receptive aphasia.

People with dysarthria also show a wide range of severity. Some have trouble producing only a few speech sounds while others can hardly be understood.

5. Why can an aphasic patient say words on certain occasions and not at other times?

Automatic expressions occasionally account for much of a patient's speech. At times someone who is otherwise unable to express himself will say something with ease, clarity, and fluency. He cannot usually repeat these expressions or words voluntarily, and we conclude, therefore, that they are elicited on an automatic basis—that is, they are uncontrolled, unexpected responses which are not in the patient's controlled inventory of responses. We call this *automatic speech*. We all use automatic speech. "Hello," "How are you," "Well I'll be darned" are typical examples. An aphasic patient who may be unable to express himself when he has a thought or an idea that he wants to convey sometimes produces automatic expressions. They are analogous to the automatic way a person drives a car. He doesn't think of moving his foot from the accelerator to the brake at the right time, he just does it.

It is easy for those close to an aphasic patient to interpret these occasional automatic expressions as signs of recovery. Unfortunately, this is not the case. As a matter of fact, the patient is usually inconsistent and if asked to repeat the automatic phrase will be unable to do so.

Another reason for inconsistency in speech is that a large proportion of stroke patients are inconsistent in many things. For example, a patient may walk much better on one day than on another or even at different times during the same day. This is one of the results of damage to the brain.

6. If an aphasic patient can sing and count why can't he speak?

Research workers have demonstrated that the appreciation and production of music and the understanding and production of speech are under the control of two entirely different parts of the brain. As a matter of fact, the speech control centers are usually in the left half of the brain and the music centers in the right half. The words that go along with music must be very closely tied to the music itself, since patients with aphasia can sing the words to songs they have known very well but will be unable to use the same words in ordinary speech.

Counting is a form of automatic speech; so is reciting the alphabet or the days of the week. They are automatic in series but cease to be automatic when they are isolated. For example, a patient may be able to count from one to ten, but if you ask him how many fingers he has on his left hand, he may not be able to tell you. Sometimes he can answer you by counting up to five.

7. Is it natural for an aphasic patient to use his native language more easily than a second language?

Yes. An aphasic patient usually finds it easier to use his native language than an acquired language. This may sometimes be true even if he hasn't used his first language for a long time. Similarly, the aphasic patient usually recovers his native language more rapidly than his second language. If it is apparent to the therapist that the patient will recover his native language more quickly, he may supervise his speech rehabilitation in that language. The principles and techniques of aphasia rehabilitation are the same in all languages.

8. Can aphasia be temporary?

In medical circles, temporary aphasia is known as *transient aphasia,* and it refers to a communication problem lasting only a few days or weeks following a stroke. More than half of the patients who initially show aphasia symptoms recover completely during the first few days. Sir Winston Churchill and the late President Eisenhower are good examples of individuals who suffered transient aphasia. Our concern in this chapter, however, is primarily with those patients whose aphasia persists after the first few days or weeks.

9. Can a patient sometimes read and write and yet not speak?

Yes. In the answer to Question 1 we described the six functions which are part of language or communication and said that any or all could be impaired after a stroke. It is possible, therefore, to see someone who can read and write but not speak, or, conversely, who can speak but not read or write. There are other combinations.

This is often difficult for the families of aphasic patients to understand because reading, writing, and speaking are so closely linked. But there are different patterns of loss, and it should never be assumed that a person can perform well in all forms of communication until he has been thoroughly tested.

10. Does a patient's speech disorder ever become worse?

In general, speech disorders resulting from strokes do not become worse. On the contrary, we generally expect an improvement with time. In the rare cases where there is noticeable deterioration, the patient's doctor should be consulted promptly.

There are times when a patient's speech is temporarily worse than it is at other times. Fatigue, depression, or emotional stress can do this, and it is easy to understand since even normal speakers experience diminished speech proficiency under conditions of stress.

11. Does the patient's difficulty in reading have anything to do with vision?

Many stroke patients have visual field defects (see Question 3, Chapter 2) which *mechanically* interfere with reading. The person with an aphasic reading impairment has a different problem that results from damage in the communication center of the brain. He will be able to see all the words; indeed, he may be able to read them aloud, but he may not understand what he is reading. This is a difficult idea to comprehend since we assume that a person who can read words must know what he's reading. But the aphasic doesn't; it is similar to reading words in a foreign language and not knowing what they mean.

12. What is the connection between eating and speech?

None, except in the patient who has dysarthria (see Question 1). Since many of the muscles used in eating are the same as those used for speaking, the patient with dysarthria may also have trouble chewing and swallowing food; he may sometimes regurgitate food, drool, or find it difficult to suck liquids through a straw. (Playing a wind instrument or whistling might be difficult, too.)

There is no similar relationship between eating and speech in the person with aphasia or verbal apraxia, because these patients have no trouble with the eating and speaking muscles. Their major difficulty is in the communication center of the brain. However, they often have weakness of the muscles of the right side of the face and loss of sensation inside the mouth on the right side, with the result that food may lodge between the teeth and cheek. Although this does not adversely affect the patient's ability to speak, members of the family are often concerned that it does.

13. I know that the patient can say a lot of things. Why doesn't he?

Whenever we discuss this subject with family members, we realize that they are usually referring to the fact that they have heard the patient use automatic expressions but then do not hear these same words in different phrases. In Question 5 it was explained that since these expressions are automatic, the words in them are not always available to the patient. Hence, his listeners think that he has more words at his command than he actually does.

In some cases patients do have more speech than they are using but speak less because they are depressed, frustrated, or ashamed of their problem. Sometimes it is simply a function of inconsistency—they do better on some days than on others. Patients frequently don't speak as well when they are being tested.

In general, these are not significant problems, and patients use every bit of residual speech they have.

14. Does the patient mean it when he swears?

Some do and some don't. There are aphasic patients who swear easily and often as a result of uncontrolled automatic speech. On the other hand, a person may swear as a direct expression of anger and frustration, and such language is appropriate to the situation in which he finds himself. The fact that a patient frequently swears is unrelated to whether or not he swore before the stroke. Sometimes he simply has a reduced ability to inhibit some of his responses, and where he would have exercised self-control before, his present condition doesn't allow him to.

In any case, family members should not become disturbed but should understand that whether the expression is automatic or not, it is a result of the patient's condition.

15. Does a stroke cause a hearing loss?

No, because there are hearing centers on both sides of the brain and the stroke only affects one side (see also Question 5, Chapter 2). However, it is easy to confuse a deficiency in understanding spoken language, which is a common characteristic of aphasia, with an impairment of hearing. To avoid this confusion the patient's hearing is tested at the time of his speech evaluation. Since many patients who have had strokes are in the middle or older age groups, some are found to have diminished hearing as part of the aging process.

It is occasionally reported by a family member that an aphasic patient seems to hear more than he did prior to his stroke. The reason for this is that his disability causes him to pay closer attention to what's going on around him. This should not be confused with an improvement in hearing.

16. Do patients understand more when the subject is familiar to them?

There is no doubt that aphasic patients understand familiar material better than they do the unfamiliar. Family members who have seen a patient being tested or treated often report that he does better at home than at the rehabilitation center. Familiar surroundings, familiar subjects, and even the private language that exists between a husband and wife make this understandable.

17. Why is it difficult for an aphasic patient to follow conversation in a crowd?

Aphasic patients frequently complain that they have a more difficult time conversing in a noisy room or with groups of people. They say it is tiring and requires great effort and concentration. Conversation with one person is usually easier.

One of the principal reasons for this is the patient's receptive or comprehension deficiency—he must try to single out the voice of the person he is listening to and is distracted by other voices and noise. He may also find it difficult to concentrate, and if he has a mild memory problem will not be able to recall all that is said by the various speakers.

Social events and receiving visitors should be carefully planned to avoid exposing the patient to what can be a very frustrating experience.

18. Is there any medicine which can cure aphasia?

No medicines, drugs, or surgery have been known to cure aphasia. Your physician may prescribe certain medications which will help the patient's physical or emotional condition. He may sleep better or his general mood may improve as a result of these medications. However, aphasia cannot be changed by medication. In view of this, one should be cautious of such claims. Above all, do not attempt to recommend or prescribe medicine yourself. If any medication is called for, your physician will prescribe it.

19. Can hypnosis cure aphasia?

No. There is no evidence that hypnosis can affect the course of recovery since aphasia is the result of injury to the brain. Hypnosis could be effective only if aphasia were a condition resulting from emotional or psychological factors.

20. Will massage or physical therapy of the vocal area help aphasia?

No. Physical treatment will not improve the patient's ability to speak. Although he may have paralysis of the right side of the face, including the right side of the mouth and tongue, this does not prevent him from speaking. The cause of aphasia is not facial paralysis, vocal cord paralysis, or injury to the "voice box."

21. What can be done to help the aphasic improve his language function?

The only direct help known for aphasia is speech therapy. It is best for the patient to receive therapy from a speech pathologist, preferably one who has had experience with stroke patients, since the communication problems following stroke are unique and require special training. Your doctor can help you locate a speech pathologist who is properly trained. They are usually on the staffs of rehabilitation centers or large hospitals.

22. How soon after the onset of aphasia should speech therapy begin?

As soon as the acute stage of illness has passed. The acute stage refers to the time when the patient is in bed and is quite sick. Once he is allowed to be up, one can think about the necessary rehabilitation measures, including speech therapy.

There are good reasons why speech therapy should be started as soon as possible. During the first six months following a stroke the damaged part of the brain is attempting to heal itself. This is known as the period of "spontaneous recovery." Experience has shown that patients do better if they receive speech therapy during this period. It should be understood, however, that much of the recovery of language depends upon the healing process in the brain. It is the speech therapist's job to see that all of the recovered language is used. Furthermore, the period immediately after a stroke is the most frightening for a person with aphasia, and there is no doubt that working with someone who understands his problem is comforting.

23. What is a speech therapist? A speech pathologist?

The correct title for those who treat aphasic patients is "speech pathologist." By common usage they are often referred to as "speech therapists." To qualify for the title of speech pathologist, one must earn a master's degree and have experience in the treatment of patients. The requirements are outlined by the American Speech and Hearing Association, and when they are fulfilled the person is granted a Certificate of Clinical Competence by that association.

Speech pathologists are trained to treat a variety of speech disorders in both children and adults. They work in private practice, university clinics, private speech and hearing clinics, rehabilitation centers, and hospitals. The American Speech and Hearing Association, which has headquarters at 9030 Old Georgetown Road, Washington, D.C., 20014, publishes a directory of speech pathologists.

24. What does the speech pathologist actually do?

The basic principle in speech therapy, as in all rehabilitation therapy, is to help the patient fully utilize all of his remaining skills. You will remember that with communication disorders this includes speaking, reading, writing, and understanding the spoken word. The way that the therapist approaches treatment is to identify those areas in which the patient does best and to start working there. For example, if the patient has no speech left at all but has some ability to write, the emphasis will be on writing for a while. One hopes that this will stimulate other language areas.

Another goal of speech therapy is to improve consistency of performance. In the case of an aphasic patient who can use a particular word 10 percent of the time, the therapist will try to make that word usable 70 or 80 percent of the time. Hence, the idea is not only to help the patient use new words and phrases, but also to enable him to use remaining language with more accuracy and consistency.

Still another important function of the speech pathologist is to explain to the patient and family what has happened in the language area and what skills the patient has left. This information is important since it helps to dispel some of the great fear which a stroke produces.

It must be borne in mind that the therapist can do no more than assist natural processes, that the real determinant of the degree of return of speech function is the healing of the damaged area of the brain.

25. What can a family do for an aphasic patient if a qualified speech pathologist is not available?

We would first suggest that every effort be made to locate a speech pathologist. If you are not near a rehabilitation center and your local hospital does not have a speech clinician,

STROKE

you can write to the American Speech and Hearing Association, 9030 Old Georgetown Road, Washington, D.C., 20014, for suggestions. Sometimes a nearby university or college will have a speech clinic.

If you cannot find a properly trained individual, then we suggest that you approach someone in the community with teaching experience. If this person is willing to help he can read this book and refer to the suggested readings under aphasia rehabilitation in the Appendix.

We have known of some families who have been unable for geographic or economic reasons to engage the help of an outsider and who have done a magnificent job of rehabilitation at home using some published materials designed for the purpose (see Appendix) and some ingenious methods of their own design.

26. How long will the patient need speech therapy?

Unfortunately this is impossible to predict. It depends on the patient's motivation, his ability to improve, and the severity of the aphasia. It is generally agreed that aphasia recovery is a long, slow process, and one must think in terms of months and years, not days and weeks. Some show progress for a period of only a few months while others change more slowly. In any event, there are very few cases on record of aphasia disappearing suddenly except in those patients with transient aphasia (see Question 8). In almost all instances, language is recovered gradually, and the most significant improvement occurs during the first six months following onset.

In view of these facts, speech therapy is usually given during the first six months following a stroke for varying periods of time. Some patients are treated for only a few weeks, some for a few months.

Unrealistic goals in aphasia rehabilitation must be avoided. It is better to set small goals to be met from week to week rather than the long-range goal of normal speech. Once a speech disorder has persisted for six months, it is not likely that normal speech will be regained. If one is reasonably sure that the patient will not recover completely, it is cruel to create false hopes. This can only lead to failure and greater depression. When speech therapy is given for longer than six months it is usually for the psychological support of the patient. It should be clearly understood by the patient and his family that although the process of language recovery may go on for a period of years, speech therapy is not indicated during all of that time.

27. How long should speech therapy sessions be?

Both the length and frequency of speech therapy sessions are determined by the patient's condition. We have learned from experience that sessions must be short since the great majority of people with aphasia fatigue very easily and have a limited attention span. As a consequence, the practice in most rehabilitation centers is to give speech therapy for thirty minutes from two to five times a week. There are deviations from this routine, but only when physician and therapist agree that it is best for the patient.

Family and friends often assume that if a little bit of therapy is good, a lot is better. As with so many things, this is simply not so.

28. Should the patient be forced to attend speech therapy?

The majority of patients with speech disorders are extremely anxious to have therapy. There is an occasional one who refuses to attend sessions; he should not be forced to it, since he will derive no benefit from therapy under those circumstances.

29. Should a family member attend speech therapy sessions with the patient?

This decision will depend on the speech therapist and the patient's physician. Generally speaking, it is advisable for the patient to be alone with the therapist during training sessions. This permits the therapist to control the situation properly, and it makes the establishment of a close relationship with the patient easier. The presence of a wife or husband may introduce pressures which shouldn't exist during a therapy session.

In some cases, however, the presence of a family member is desirable. This holds if the relative is participating in supplementary training at home or if it is necessary to demonstrate what progress the patient is or is not making. In all cases the decision to include a family member is a clinical one and must be made by the therapist or physician.

30. Is there group speech therapy?

The group technique is usually used for social and psychological reasons, since it provides aphasic patients the opportunity to use speech in a social setting—an opportunity they may not otherwise have. Also, some patients derive psychological benefit from associating with others who are aphasic. Group therapy is not available in all centers, in some it is the only method of speech therapy, and in others it supplements individual speech therapy sessions.

31. Why not teach the aphasic patient a substitute language?

The idea of finding a substitute language for the aphasic patient has tempted both laymen and professionals for a long time. Some of the common questions are "Why can't you teach the patient a hand sign language?" or "Why can't he be taught to use a typewriter for communication?" We have heard these and many other similar suggestions.

The problem is that the very same factors which prevent the patient from speaking and writing also prevent him from learning to use a new language system. One of the proofs of this is that congenitally deaf people who use sign language may lose it when they have a stroke, and secretaries who have a stroke often lose the ability to take shorthand. In other words, the person who would have the capacity to learn sign language would also be able to speak and write. If he has aphasia it extends to all types of communication including any that we might devise for him. This is the great tragedy of aphasia. To answer the other question, the use of a typewriter is basically no different from writing. When we write we form letters into words, words into phrases, and phrases into sentences. And when we type we do precisely the same thing. A patient who cannot write a sentence cannot type a sentence.

We understand the tremendous desire of family and friends to find some way of helping a person with aphasia. Unfortunately, substitute languages cannot do this. We are consoled by the fact that in time patients do find ways to communicate. We can be most helpful to them in this process by being understanding and patient.

32. What kinds of words do aphasic patients recover first?

Patients usually recover the elements of language in the followering order: nouns, verbs, adjectives, and adverbs; and finally, articles, prepositions, and conjunctions.

Many complain that they can read, write, and say everything but the "small words." This is easy to understand since the small words, the prepositions, conjunctions, and articles are usually the last ones to be recovered.

The person with aphasia generally finds it easier to use nouns since they refer to things that he can see, feel, or hear. Words such as *book, table, radio,* and *telephone* are more specific and real than words like *it, but, be, even, of,* or *for.*

33. What specific words does the therapist concentrate on at the beginning of speech therapy?

The selection of words in the first stages of aphasia rehabilitation is governed by the following criteria:

1. How important will the words be to the patient? They should apply to his immediate situation and his most essential needs such as eating, using the toilet, and dressing. For example, a patient would obviously have much more use for the word *bed* than the words *rock* or *slippery.*

2. How specific or real will the words be to the patient? As mentioned in the answer to the previous question, an aphasic patient finds it much easier to learn the names of things he can see, feel, or hear. The word *hat,* for example, is easier than the word *fear.* Although the words *food* and *clothes* seem good choices, they probably should not be included among the very first words. Both *food* and *clothes* are collective nouns, and aphasics often have difficulty dealing with the concept of collectivity.

3. How frequently are the words used in everyday communication? It would be better, for example, to select the word *mistake* rather than the word *error,* the word *house* rather than *domicile.* While *error* and *domicile* have the same meaning as *mistake* and *house,* they are used much less frequently.

After the patient has acquired a small, basic vocabulary, a

more individualized list can be presented. This list should include words of special interest to the patient. In the case of a tailor, for example, words like *needle, thread,* and *seam* would be more important and stimulating than a general word list.

Using the criteria given above, a practical and typical list of twenty-five words with which to start might include: *bed, chair, toilet, water, cigarette, coffee, money, clock, pen, telephone, doctor, shoe, car, mouth, key, soap, hand, leg, table, toothbrush, man, sandwich, house, book, cup.* Of course the list would vary from patient to patient. The word *cigarette,* for example, would not be important to a nonsmoker.

34. Should a patient with aphasia be taught how to make vowel and consonant sounds?

This is determined by the speech pathologist at the time of evaluation and depends upon the kind of speech disorder. Those who need this kind of training are patients with verbal apraxia and dysarthria, conditions which were described in Questions 1 and 2. As you will recall, these patients have problems with control of the speech muscles and therefore need training in making the sounds of speech. The patient who has only aphasia does not require such training.

It is clear from the foregoing that an accurate diagnosis of the patient's communication problem is necessary before therapy is begun. This is one of the main reasons why the services of a speech pathologist are so essential.

35. When do you start to work on reading and writing?

Reading and writing may be the first things to be taken up, or the last. It depends entirely upon how much the patient is impaired in the various language areas. If, for example, he cannot speak at all but has retained a good bit of his ability to write, the therapist will concentrate on this first. As we have said earlier, one tries to help the patient fully utilize all of the skills which he has left. Experience has shown that the best results are obtained by working first with those modalities which are strongest. The patient's therapist is best qualified to make these decisions.

36. Why does the speech therapist train the patient to write with his left hand?

A right-handed person will be taught to use his right hand for writing if possible. However, most people with aphasia also have weakness or paralysis of the right hand and must be taught to use the left. If the right side recovers sufficiently, it can be used once again.

One point sometimes arises which should be clarified. The speech therapist is not concerned with making the patient's handwriting esthetically acceptable, regardless of which hand is used. He is simply trying to develop this means of communication as fully as possible.

37. Should the patient be taught to print or to write words?

This decision should be left to the patient since he usually has a preference, and it makes no difference to his recovery.

38. The speech therapist seems to use childish methods. Is this necessary?

Elementary methods are often necessary in the course of therapy. This reflects the degree of language impairment and is *not* a measure of the patient's intelligence. We have had patients of very high intelligence who were able to think as well after the stroke as before. But they, too, required the use of simple materials because, though the thinking apparatus was normal, language function was severely damaged. It goes without saying that as the patient recovers the therapist will use more sophisticated material.

39. Does the patient know he has aphasia?

Yes. Except for the rare individual whose stroke is so severe that he doesn't know who he is or where he is, the patient always knows he has a speech disorder. He is immediately aware of even the slightest change in his ability to talk or understand the spoken word. He may not discover that he has trouble with reading and writing until quite a while after the stroke, because these are usually not tried during the first few weeks.

Some aphasic patients who use jargon are not aware of the fact that their speech may be meaningless.

40. Should a patient be told that he has aphasia?

No one needs to tell a patient that he is having trouble with his speech or any of the other communication modalities—he knows it very well. And he is sure to be depressed and extremely frightened at what has happened. What he needs is an explanation by a doctor or a speech pathologist as to what has happened in terms he can understand, for knowing some of the details of his condition can help reduce his anxiety.

41. Do aphasic patients sometimes look at newspapers even though they have a reading impairment?

Yes. Many continue to look at newspapers even though they don't understand everything they're reading. This is probably a carry-over from the habit of newspaper reading. However, the speech therapist can usually determine just how much reading a patient can do. Even though he may understand little, his interest in looking at newspapers should not be discouraged.

42. Do aphasic patients have difficulty concentrating when reading?

Many patients complain that they can no longer concentrate on reading even though they may be interested and able to understand what they read. This should not be considered a negative sign. A patient's ability to concentrate almost always improves with time. At first, he may be able to concentrate on only one page of a book per sitting. If he continues to read for short, frequent periods each day, his ability to concentrate may be expected to improve.

Sometimes an aphasic patient's difficulty in reading is related to a problem in retaining (or remembering) what he has read. This problem is very different from concentrating on what is being read.

43. Does a patient with aphasia have a shortened attention span?

This is a fairly common problem for the aphasic patient, and if he has it he may have trouble sticking to a task long enough to complete it. He may also be easily distracted by noises and interruptions. This shortened attention span and easy distractibility can interfere considerably with a patient's ability to make progress in a rehabilitation program.

Some aphasic patients also have difficulty retaining information. A word seemingly acquired at one moment may be lost in the next. Attention span and retention are factors which can retard a patient's ability to improve with speech therapy.

100

44. Does aphasia have anything to do with mental illness?

Disorders in speech, reading, or writing have nothing to do with mental incompetence. These are separate functions of the brain and should not be confused. An occasional patient with a communication problem may also have some difficulty in his thinking capacity, but the two are not related.

Mental illness to most people means that the person has a psychiatric condition. Again, there is no relationship between such conditions and speech disorders because they represent different functions of the brain. This is an important point since the families and friends of patients with aphasia worry about this and frequently assume that because a person has a speech disorder there must be something wrong with him mentally, either in the thinking or the psychiatric sense.

It is true that some patients with aphasia act differently for a while (this is discussed more fully in Chapter 4), but many of them have the same mental and emotional capacities they had prior to the stroke.

45. How can I tell how much the patient really knows or thinks?

It is sometimes difficult when an individual has limited skill in communication to determine how much he actually knows. Since it is not possible to look into the brain, estimates of how much a person thinks or knows must be based on his actions and whatever residual gestures he possesses.

Attempts to read a patient's facial expression to get an idea of what he's thinking are often misleading. Facial expressions may reflect a mood rather than specific information. On the other hand, families and others close to a patient can often read his expressions since they know his likes, dislikes, feelings, and opinions.

46. Is a patient with aphasia capable of knowing what time it is?

Knowing what time it is—called "time orientation"—is not necessarily impaired in aphasic patients. The fact that the patient can't tell you the time doesn't mean that he doesn't *know* what time it is. As a matter of fact, some patients with aphasia become preoccupied with time and rigid about adhering to their daily time schedules. They are very often upset if a therapy session starts a few minutes late, if breakfast isn't served at the designated time, or if a visitor doesn't arrive precisely on time.

47. Should a patient with a speech disorder be discouraged from associating with other patients with speech problems?

Sometimes families are afraid that the patient's communication difficulties will worsen if he is in contact with other aphasic patients, or that he will not be stimulated to talk in such a situation. This idea has often led to the request that the patient not share a room in the hospital with other aphasics.

Actually most aphasic patients enjoy each other's company. They undoubtedly derive comfort from associating with others who share a similar disability and face the same kinds of problems. Contrary to what one might expect, they have a remarkable facility for communicating with each other no matter how severely impaired they may be. There is a lot to be said for the understanding that can be shared only by those who find themselves in the same situation after a catastrophic illness or event.

48. Is it possible for a patient to become too dependent on the use of gestures?

The person who has a speech problem is justified in using any means of communication he can. We believe that in the great majority of patients the desire to speak is so strong that they will do so if they possibly can. If someone resorts to the use of gestures, even a great deal of the time, it means that he must do so in order to express himself; this should not be discouraged. Gestures are an excellent substitution for speech, and it's not valid to say that someone may become too dependent on them.

49. How long should you wait for an aphasic patient to answer a question?

There is no specific answer to this question since the appropriate waiting time will depend on the situation and will vary from person to person. Naturally one should give an aphasic patient more than the average amount of time to respond. On the other hand waiting too long while he struggles with an answer can be very frustrating for him. If he is showing frustration and irritation over his inability to respond, it is sometimes best simply to suggest that he wait and try again later.

What is most important is that you avoid becoming anxious about the slowness of his responses. You can never be really wrong if you reassure him by remaining calm and conducting your interaction with him in a matter-of-fact way.

50. How should one talk to a person who has aphasia?

We have had this question put to us hundreds of times and believe that it must arise in the mind of everyone who lives

103

with a person suffering from aphasia. Following are the guidelines we would suggest.

First, it is a good idea to talk a little slower than usual since the patient may have a problem understanding rapid speech and will need the extra time to figure out what's being said.

Then, one must be sure not to talk loudly; we all tend to do this because we think the patient can't hear so well when, in fact, there's usually nothing wrong with his hearing.

It is a good idea to use simple words and simple phrases. Don't change the melody of your speech; by this we mean that your inflections should be the same as they usually are because the aphasic depends upon this.

Don't overtalk. This is usually a result of one's own anxiety and may be transmitted to the patient. Further, this will make it difficult for him to express himself since he won't be able to break into the flow of your conversation.

When talking to someone who has no speech at all, it is suggested that questions be put in such a way that they can be answered with "yes" or "no." For example, rather than ask "Where would you like to go tonight?" say "Would you like to go to the movies tonight?"

Finally, it is most important not to talk to him as if he were a child. This is one of the easiest and most frequent pitfalls. We have said elsewhere that the patient is not retarded. On the contrary, in most cases his intellect is completely intact, and it is most demoralizing to be spoken to as a child.

51. Should I let the patient know that I don't understand him?

It makes little sense to pretend to understand what the patient is saying. This technique solves nothing and may contribute to a great deal of misunderstanding. Actually, most patients are aware that they are not being understood and become irritated with those around them who behave as if they did. If you are honest and use common sense, you won't get into trouble.

52. Why does the patient say "yes" to some questions when it's obvious he doesn't understand them?

As a matter of fact, all of us are guilty of this at one time or another because we don't want the person with whom we're talking to know that we didn't understand. This is particularly true of people with aphasia. In fact, some will talk incessantly to avoid having you ask them a question. Over and over we must remind ourselves how devastating it is to a person to lose any of his language faculties.

53. The patient talks all the time; a lot of it I can't understand. What is this?

People with aphasia usually speak very little because their vocabularies are small. Some, however, talk continuously despite a reduced vocabulary; this is generally due to anxiety.

The type of patient to whom this questioner refers has what we have previously described as jargon (see Question 3). His speech is unintelligible for the most part, and he may use a great deal of expression as though he were really communicating an idea. Occasionally, he will intersperse the jargon with real words. It is difficult to tell whether such patients are aware that they haven't been understood, for sometimes they will show frustration or be irritated with the listener.

This situation can be very upsetting to family members. They struggle to understand the jargon, may become irritated by their inability to do so, and sometimes become angry at the patient. One must bear in mind that he has no control over this phenomenon, and that there is little one can do to change it. Fortunately, jargon may decrease or disappear as a patient recovers language.

54. Can you give me some good ideas on how I can understand someone who has very little speech?

Over and over again we are gratified to see how a husband and wife learn to communicate with each other despite the fact that one of them has very little speech. At the beginning it seems like an almost impossible task, but that's because they're so unaccustomed to it. In essence, the idea is to play the game of twenty questions. By mentioning all of the possibilities that the patient might be trying to communicate, you can eventually narrow it down to the correct one. He, on his part, must play the game of charades and learn to use his power of gesturing fully.

55. Should I correct the patient?

This question cannot be answered categorically, but we would say, in general, no. The reason is that the aphasic patient is not making mistakes out of stupidity, stubbornness, or perversity. He has problems with his speech which are not under his control. To correct him serves no purpose, since he will correct himself if he can. And if he can't, no amount of suggestion from anyone else will help. Furthermore, correcting an aphasic perpetuates the tendency to deal with him like a child, and this is to be avoided under all circumstances. This also tends to make him angry and sometimes anxious.

56. Does it help to speak to the patient on his unaffected side?

Sometimes, though not frequently, a patient will understand more of what is said if the speaker addresses him on his unaffected side. We don't understand this, but if you have observed that it is true by all means do it. There are many mysteries in aphasia, and this is one of them.

57. Should a person with aphasia be encouraged or discouraged to use the telephone?

He should be neither discouraged nor encouraged. The decision is up to the patient who knows his own limitations and the strength of his motivation.

Once a patient has decided to make a call, you can be of assistance by remembering the following things. Dialing a telephone requires the use of numbers, and the patient may have a number problem. In many areas of the United States the telephone company has a system which makes dialing possible for such people. It is called the Card Dialer. A card containing the name or picture of someone who is frequently called is punched with the person's telephone number. By dropping the card into a slot on a special telephone, the desired number is automatically dialed.

For patients who have great difficulty expressing themselves, friends and relatives should be forewarned to do most of the talking and to ask questions to which the patient can respond with "yes" or "no."

Families have reported that aphasic patients speak better on the telephone than in face-to-face conversation. We have not observed this, but if it occurs it may be because the patient does not see the person with whom he is talking; he is not directly confronted by someone, and this may make it easier for him. Also, it is possible that he is less distracted by noises in the room, other people talking, etc., when speaking on the telephone.

58. Why doesn't the patient read or play cards anymore when he used to enjoy these activities?

First, let us deal with the question of reading. It is obvious that if a person's reading is impaired, it will no longer be available to him as a pastime. However, some people can still read very well but don't. This may be due to decreased attention span or simply because of generalized anxiety. (We have found this to hold true for other activities.) Certain patients continue to read for pleasure but will read only magazines and newspapers.

Do not try to get the patient to play word games like scrabble or to do crossword puzzles. Families often conclude that if the patient's trouble is with words such games must obviously benefit him. Actually, the reverse is true, since such games inevitably prove to be frustrating to the patient.

Playing cards, chess, and checkers seems to be a different matter, for most aphasic patients can play these games if they did before. This is because they have very little to do with language.

Other pastimes which do not require language skill and which many aphasics enjoy include jigsaw puzzles, painting, sculpture, listening to music, gardening, and fishing. It must be said, however, that introducing new activities to aphasic patients is generally very difficult.

If one is looking for a guiding principle in all of this, it should be that one must try to stimulate the person's interest in something. This may be a difficult task, as anyone knows who has tried to get an elderly person to become active again. The physical and psychological effort seem just too great for many of these people. However, we have seen such people take interest and take heart once more.

59. Will the patient's aphasia improve as his physical condition improves?

Improvement in language skill does not necessarily accompany improvement in physical condition; the two areas must be considered independently. Some aphasic patients have *no* physical disabilities. In general, however, language skills take longer to recover than physical skills. For example, the patient will usually learn to walk before he learns to talk. There is no hard and fast rule to the order of recovery since this depends entirely on the area and extent of injury to the brain.

60. I heard of someone who woke up speaking normally a year after his stroke. Is this possible?

This type of question is commonly asked and springs from the intense desire for a cure, particularly if it can be miraculous. Unfortunately, the lay press occasionally prints stories of prominent people who had aphasia and recovered completely, implying that this can happen to anyone if he receives the best care. The fact is that no two cases are exactly alike, and before making comparisons one must know the details. Further, the extent of recovery is not dependent upon treatment but on the degree of healing which occurs in the brain. The prince and the pauper have the same chance for recovery. One must listen to stories of miraculous cures with healthy skepticism.

In those rare cases in which the patient begins to talk after being totally mute for a year, one can be sure that the mutism was not caused by aphasia or dysarthria. It is possible that the patient was so severely depressed that he refused to talk. This is rare, and, as a matter of fact, in many years of experience we have never seen it.

The important thing to remember is that there are trained professionals who are experienced in diagnosing speech disorders and who know what the usual course of recovery is. Those who work with aphasic patients are just as anxious as members of the family to see them recover and can help develop a realistic appraisal of the patient's prospects for recovery.

61. Is it possible for an aphasic patient to recover more language two or three years after the onset of the stroke?

It is possible but very unlikely that a patient will make any dramatic improvement in language many years after the onset of the stroke. The greatest and most obvious improvement occurs during the first six months. After this, they generally continue to make small, gradual gains for an indefinite period.

In certain cases of verbal apraxia (see Questions 1 and 2), one may see substantial improvement over a longer period of time than in those patients whose primary problem is aphasia.

62. Will a patient improve after he stops speech therapy?

Many patients continue to improve without help long after they have terminated speech treatment. As mentioned before, however, the changes that occur after the first few months are usually very gradual and subtle.

63. Does the patient's speech become normal again?

Unless recovery occurs during the first few weeks, very few aphasic patients regain completely normal use of language. Even in those cases where the result seems to be "normal," careful testing will usually reveal that there are still mild deficiencies. Happily, they do not interfere with everyday communication and are barely perceptible.

64. Will the aphasic patient be able to return to his previous job?

There are many variables that must be considered when making this decision. Among the more important of these is the personality of the patient and his reaction to having aphasia. Some would not return to work under any circumstances even if only a mild speech disorder remained. These are the patients who are extremely sensitive about not being "normal." Those who can go back have either conquered this sensitivity or never had it to begin with.

What is probably of greatest importance is the type and severity of the speech disorder and the language requirements of the job. Remember that this includes speaking, understanding the spoken word, reading, writing, and calculation, any or all of which may be involved. Most of us don't realize how important these language skills are in almost all vocations. A plumber must answer the telephone, speak to his customers, read instructions, write orders, submit bills, etc. Clerical workers and professionals, who use language skills even more, are the hardest hit and are frequently disappointed when they try to return to the job.

Fortunately, most patients know better than their advisors what they can and cannot do; they know better than anyone else the demands of their jobs and whether or not they can fulfill them. It is the desire of a family member to know as soon as possible the answers to questions such as, "Shall we keep a law office open, shall we hire an associate, shall we sell the business?" These are typical concerns. Until the outcome is clear, which may mean a year or so after onset, the answer must be deferred and a holding operation is suggested.

65. What progress has been made in treating aphasia and is there research going on?

The field of aphasia rehabilitation is very young and dates back only to World War II. While we cannot claim any startling breakthrough in the solution of this complex problem, a great deal has been accomplished during this brief time.

As a result of the development of various tests, we are now better able to identify the type and severity of speech disorders and to measure progress. Currently, speech pathologists are experimenting with treatment methods from other fields such as programmed instruction, operant conditioning, and reinforcement techniques. All of this plus considerable accumulated experience with conventional methods are improving standards of treatment.

Another measure of progress in the field is the larger number of people who are becoming interested in aphasia. Many graduate programs in speech pathology now offer special courses in aphasia. Both the government and private foundations are allocating more money every year for training and research in the field.

One of the most interesting and indicative developments in recent years has been the formation of the Academy of Aphasia. Composed of speech pathologists, speech scientists, linguists, psychologists, and physicians, this group is dedicated to the study of all aspects of the problem of aphasia.

CHAPTER 4

The Intellectual and Emotional Aspects of Stroke

1. Does a stroke affect the mind?
2. What is coma and what does it mean if a stroke starts that way?
3. What is amnesia? Does someone with a stroke have it?
4. Does the patient's personality change after a stroke?
5. What does the patient feel like after a stroke?
6. Should a patient be told what has happened to him?
7. What does it do to the patient who knows he is no longer the "boss" or breadwinner in his family?
8. Why can't the patient accept his stroke?
9. Why is the patient depressed?
10. Why is the patient more depressed on Saturdays and Sundays?
11. Why are patients in a better mood when they're busy, receiving therapy, or with friends rather than family?
12. Does a patient get depressed when he sees other stroke patients?
13. Why does the stroke patient cry so easily?

14. Why does the patient sometimes laugh inappropriately?
15. Why does the patient sometimes act childish?
16. Why are patients sometimes aggressive when they never were before?
17. Why does the patient lose his temper and shout now when he never did before?
18. Why do stroke patients sometimes get fixed on unimportant things?
19. The patient doesn't seem to be able to concentrate on anything for long. Why not?
20. Why does the patient refuse to go out?
21. If the patient was considerate before, will he be after a stroke?
22. Does the patient know his own limitations?
23. How should I treat the patient?
24. How much should I do for the patient?
25. Should the patient be reprimanded when he is rude to other patients or friends?
26. What does one do if the patient is disinhibited in public?
27. Should business problems be discussed with a patient?
28. Should a patient be told bad news, such as the death of a relative?
29. Should I try to get the patient's mind off himself and onto my troubles?
30. Should I encourage the patient by telling him he'll be back at his old job soon?
31. Why don't our friends come to visit anymore?
32. Should I encourage friends and relatives to visit?
33. What about sexual relationships?
34. Do family relationships change after someone has had a stroke?
35. People don't realize what the family has to go through

when someone has had a stroke. Should there be some consideration for family members?

36. Is it natural to become impatient or intolerant of someone who has had a stroke?
37. Should a patient go back to a tense business?
38. Do people with strokes need to see a psychiatrist?

Introduction

The purpose of this chapter is to explain the possible effects of a stroke on a patient's thinking capacities and emotional reactions. We say "possible effects" because not everyone who sustains a stroke will experience these things. Since the degree of loss or change of function depends on the part of the brain involved and the severity of the stroke, there are great differences among patients. As we describe the various changes, it should not be assumed that every stroke patient will exhibit these changes.

It is also important to bear in mind that many of the phenomena to be described are only temporary. Whenever damage occurs to any part of the body there are certain reactions in the local area of damage which may temporarily cause more symptoms. One of these is the accumulation of fluid in and around injured tissue (*edema*). As the fluid gradually disappears, some of the symptoms which were present at first may disappear as well. Sometimes this process takes many weeks.

Finally, not all of the brain tissue involved in a stroke is permanently damaged. Some of it is only injured. As the body's healing processes go on, these injured cells recover, and there is concomitant recovery of function. This period of spontaneous healing, too, goes on for weeks.

In order to understand why a stroke may cause the damage it does, one must first understand how the brain works and how it controls mental and physical functions.

For our purposes let us think of the brain as a control and processing center. Figure 4–1 below gives most of its important functions.

The items below the dotted line are functions which the human brain has in common with lower animals. The eyes see, the ears hear, and the nose smells, but the brain interprets all of these so they have meaning. Similarly it interprets body sensations so that we automatically know where all the body parts are, whether anything painful or harmful is going on, and so on. It has partial control over certain internal organs and complete control over all movements of the head, trunk, and limbs.

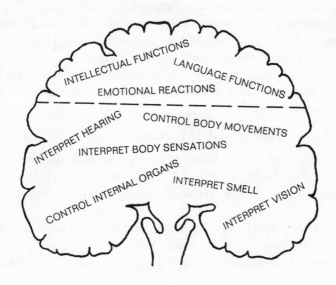

CONTROL CENTERS IN THE BRAIN

FIGURE 4–1

But it is the items above the dotted line which distinguish us from the lower animals. Although we know that some animals think and most have primitive emotional reactions, like fear, none of them thinks and feels as humans do and, of course, none can speak.

We are so accustomed to thinking and talking that most of us never wonder how the brain accomplishes these things and probably never would were it not for occurrences like stroke or head injury. When something happens to interfere with these vital human functions, we become acutely aware of them and, quite naturally, terribly frightened.

Scientists are still trying to solve the puzzle of exactly how the brain works. However, by studying what human beings do, how they react, how they learn, how they think—all of the activities known as "behavior"—we have a general idea of how the brain functions and even know, more or less, what parts of it control the different kinds of behavior.

This chapter is devoted to questions about the intellectual and emotional changes which may result from a stroke.

1. Does a stroke affect the mind?

Rather than talk of the mind, it is more accurate to refer to the intellectual and emotional functions of the brain. In certain instances one or both of these functions may be impaired.

The word "intellectual" is used here to refer to many of the highest functions of the brain. Following are descriptions of some of these functions and the changes which may occur with a stroke.

1. Abstract thinking. This is the ability to reason, to solve problems. It is called abstract as opposed to concrete thinking since it involves the use of imagination; it enables a person to read or hear an idea, think about it, and arrive at conclusions. (There are many other types of abstract reasoning.)

For example, a person employs abstract reasoning when he thinks about religion or philosophy or politics. Figuring out how to throw a party that will be successful, how to succeed on a new job, or what baseball team is going to win the World Series—all these require abstract thinking. On the other hand, taking a motor apart and putting it back together again, giving someone directions to the post office, and buying a baby carriage are all tasks that require concrete thinking to a large extent.

Abstract reasoning may be impaired for a while after a stroke. When asked to enumerate the cause of fires, the patient might say "matches" instead of carelessness, neglect, arson, defective equipment, and so on. This does not happen to all stroke patients, and in those to whom it does occur it may be mild. Friends and relatives may be aware of it, but the patient usually is not. Fortunately, in the majority of cases it improves with time. It is statistically more frequent in patients whose strokes involve the left side of the body.

2. *Judgment.* This is closely related to abstract thinking because one must be able to reason to arrive at good judgments. However, we designate it as a separate entity because faulty judgment is fairly easy to identify and is an indication that thinking processes have been impaired. Judgment problems usually occur along with reasoning impairments and parallel them in severity and persistence. A patient with poor judgment might try to stand up repeatedly despite the fact that his leg was not yet strong enough, and he had been warned of the consequences.

3. *Memory.* This requires no definition. What may not be universally known is that there are different kinds of memory, and there may be selective impairments after a stroke. It has been observed, for example, that a patient does not recall recent events but may remember things that happened thirty years ago. This is quite common.

Another distinction is made between the remembrance of things heard as opposed to those seen, so-called auditory versus visual memory. One, both, or neither may be damaged after a stroke. Sometimes the only evidence of a memory loss is the patient's inability to recall proper names.

We must warn against one pitfall—the possible confusion between memory loss and aphasia. The patient with the latter usually has no memory problem. He is blocked in the ability to *say* a word, phrase, or sentence though he may remember it perfectly well. This is explained in greater detail in Chapter 3.

4. Orientation for time, place, and person. This is a function of the brain which is easy to take for granted, since it is quite basic to know the time, where one is, and who one is. These are not lost after a stroke, but there may be some confusion in the patient's mind about them. He may not know the correct month or date or perhaps not be sure of where he is. This rarely persists beyond the first few weeks and is no cause for alarm.

5. Perception. The things one sees, hears, or touches have no meaning until they are "processed" by the brain. The image of a house strikes the retina of the eye as a meaningless group of lines, colors, and shapes which are then sent as messages to a part of the brain which actually *sees* the house. However, for the complete meaning of the house to be understood—the relationships of all the parts to each other, the entire shape, and so on—still another part of the brain must participate. This brain function is called *perception*.

Perceptual losses are usually very subtle and neither the patient nor his family are aware of them. Such things as correctly seeing the dimensions or shape of things or the accurate estimate of distances may be impaired. The patient may be unable to see a vertical line as straight up and down or to distinguish foreground from background. Dressing may be difficult because of a confusion of right and left.

Here again, there is variation from patient to patient, and many have no such problems. When these problems do

120

occur, they are rarely so severe as to interfere with daily activities, but their nuisance value may be great.

Let us now turn to another vital brain function—that which has to do with the emotions. A person is born with certain basic personality traits. As he grows and has experiences, his personality gradually develops further. By the time he is five or six years of age, the basic personality is formed, and from then on he will react to life in a way which is characteristic of his personality.

Personality, therefore, is the sum total of a person's emotions, attitudes, feelings, ways of thinking, philosophy of life, values, and so on. A thirty-year-old man doesn't react the same as a five-year-old child, but the basic traits which determine his reactions are established at a very early age.

Though people's personalities differ, they have many emotional reactions in common. This is well illustrated in people who have had strokes. Most of the succeeding questions in this chapter have to do with the emotional reactions of the patient and his family.

The question originally posed was "Does a stroke affect the mind?" It is clear from the foregoing that it may, in certain ways. However, it does not cause mental illness or mental retardation, and the patient with a stroke has not "lost his mind."

2. What is coma and what does it mean if a stroke starts that way?

Although there are certain technical differences, coma is very much like a deep sleep. All brain functions drop down to a very low level, although an electroencephalogram (brain-wave test) would continue to show activity of brain cells.

If a stroke begins with coma, it indicates that there has been a rather severe vascular accident, and the cause of it must be determined very quickly. However, it does not mean that the prognosis for recovery is necessarily bad. There are many people whose strokes start with coma and who recover completely or nearly so.

While in coma, just as when sleeping deeply, the person has no awareness, hears nothing, feels nothing. Although the situation may be serious, the patient is not aware of its gravity.

3. What is amnesia? Does someone with a stroke have it?

Amnesia is the total loss of memory for a certain period of time, and stroke patients rarely experience it. Of course, if someone is in coma he is amnesic for the time he was asleep.

It is much more common for someone to have amnesia after a head injury such as may be suffered from a blow or automobile accident.

What is often confused with amnesia is the loss of memory a patient may have after a stroke.

4. Does the patient's personality change after a stroke?

There are many personality changes in someone who has had a stroke, but fortunately they may not be permanent. This is because it is very difficult to change something as basic as personality. However, personality is composed of so many things it would be illogical not to expect at least temporary changes after a stroke. By personality we mean how someone thinks, how he reacts, how he feels about himself and the world about him. The personality is really the sum total of the nonphysical person.

In the early weeks of a stroke, personality changes may be profound. We recall a woman who said that the most difficult and frightening thing she experienced after her husband had a stroke was that she felt he was no longer the same man she had lived with and loved for forty years. What was most frightening to her was that she believed this was the way he would remain. Of course, he did not. Although he continued to have trouble with his speech and the function of his right arm and leg, it was not long before he was himself again, and they could resume the good life the stroke had interrupted.

Many of the questions which follow deal with this subject of personality changes. Some of the most striking are the tendency to depression, the withdrawal from contact with people, inappropriate laughing or crying, impatience, lack of inhibition, childishness, lack of initiative. Not all patients show all of these, and in most people there is a tendency to return to what they were before.

5. What does the patient feel like after a stroke?

The preceding question dealt with the personality changes which someone on the outside observes in the person who does not recover quickly from a stroke. Another part of the same thing, the most important aspect, is how the patient feels.

Knowledge about this comes from conversation with hundreds of patients and from the accounts of professional writers like Eric Hodgins and Guy Wint who have had strokes.* It is important for those of us who live or work with patients to understand what is going on inside of them so that we can be more helpful and more patient.

Many patients experience fear during the early days, although some have a kind of indifference which precludes this fear.

Depression is almost universal. The patient has no desire to be with people, partially from indifference, but also be-

* See Appendix for books by these writers.

cause of shame over his altered state. Some patients report feeling no anxiety about their families, financial matters, their jobs, etc. Almost all patients are irritated by noises; they find crowds intolerable and avoid them. Many say that they have no energy, and they try to avoid activity, particularly anything which requires intense effort. In other words they feel a general lassitude which is extremely difficult to overcome. At the same time there may be an element of mental unrest.

Another feeling which the patient frequently expresses is that he is no longer part of the world's activities, that he is isolated and detached. Extremely common is the complaint that life has no zest or flavor, that everything is grey and uninteresting.

Perhaps one of the most poignant of feelings is the patient's hope that he will recover completely. Even in the most intelligent patient, this may persist long after the likelihood of full recovery is gone. Guy Wint said, "Even while hoping I was ashamed of my hope, but I hoped nevertheless."

One could not possibly detail all of the patient's reactions and sensations after a stroke. These are a few of the most striking and frequent; some of them are subjects of later questions.

6. Should a patient be told what has happened to him?

Hopefully, we are emerging from the era when having certain diseases bears a social stigma. Tuberculosis, cancer, and stroke have been such diseases. Heart disease has always been respectable. Of course, we realize that there should be no shame attached to having any disease unless it be the shame that society must bear for allowing preventable diseases to occur.

You will do the stroke patient no harm by telling him what has happened. You may, in fact, do him good if you see to it that he learns what a stroke is and how it occurs. Knowledge has a way of dispelling fear, an old truism that is no less true for the stroke patient.

Not to tell the patient is to treat him as a child. Having a stroke or any other disabling condition is a blow to a person's self-esteem, and treating him as a child only intensifies his feelings of worthlessness. Furthermore, a matter-of-fact approach to the problem will help to dispel some of the shame.

7. What does it do to the patient who knows he is no longer the "boss" or breadwinner in his family?

This question does not apply to those patients who get better within a few weeks after a stroke. In the absence of a quick and full recovery, however, the patient may have very disturbing feelings about himself. Let us see why.

Deep within the recesses of the mind each one of us has built up an image of himself over the years. One hears a great deal about people's images these days—public figures are very concerned about them so that people will like them, vote for them, or go see them in a show. We are all alike in this respect—we want the image to be a good one so that we will feel comfortable about ourselves and so that other people will like and respect us.

But this image, the one we have in our minds, is usually composed of many parts. For example, a man may be proud of his physique or of his athletic prowess; he may be proud that he is the "boss" and breadwinner in his house, that he has an important job. At the same time he may be worried about the fact that he doesn't have enough nerve to ask his boss for a raise, that he can't hold an intelligent conversation about jazz, or that he has a short temper.

So the image a person has of himself is usually composed of some things of which he is proud and some of which he is ashamed. Sometimes people are not even aware of some of the elements of their images. In any case, the good and the bad parts are usually in a kind of balance, and the person who goes through life feeling generally good about himself has more positive elements in his self-image than negative ones.

Then he has a stroke and immediately the balance changes. Some of the things about which he felt proud before are taken away from him. Suddenly he's no longer "boss" or breadwinner, can't walk or play handball, perhaps can't even dress himself. At that moment it matters not to him whether he will recover or even how much of the positive image is still there. The scales have been tipped, the balanced changed—now the feelings of inferiority (which are a part of almost everyone's self-image) are stronger than the good feelings.

This happens to everyone with a stroke. The housewife temporarily loses her role as homemaker and perhaps as mother. Grandfather can no longer go out and beat his cronies at checkers, and Aunt Matilda can't attend the Golden Age Club meetings.

These are tremendously difficult things for people to face, and those who live with a stroke patient must show him that they understand what he is going through and emphasize to him that many of the positive parts of his image are still intact.

8. Why can't the patient accept his stroke?

One might also ask, who could? Actually, the term "accept his stroke" is a poor one, for no one in his right mind would "accept" such a thing. It is more accurate to talk about how the person *reacts* to his stroke, and what we usually mean is that he is reacting to it very poorly. But this is easy to understand if one considers what the loss of speech or the use of an arm or leg can mean to a person, even if it is only temporary.

First, there is the blow to his self-image, which was described in the preceding answer. The consequences of this are feelings of shame and inferiority. We are all to blame for this because it is part of our culture to look with disapproval on anyone who is different—in size, in color, in religion, in customs, and, as in this case, in the condition of the body.

Then there are the changes which occur in someone's life pattern, as with any serious illness. Strokes usually occur in older people who have worked hard all their lives and developed a way of living which is pleasing to them. This may be interrupted or permanently changed.

And then the all-pervading fear that accompanies a stroke: fear of disability, fear of dependence, fear of the future. Taking all this into account, is it any wonder that the stroke patient reacts to his illness with depression, anger, or withdrawal, or that he is unable to "accept" it with equanimity or good grace?

Those of us who live or work with the patient must try to understand what he feels, let him know that we understand, and gently help him to overcome these feelings. It is a job requiring patience and perseverance, but for both the patient and his friends and relatives, it is preferable to sitting and wringing one's hands in despair and frustration.

9. Why is the patient depressed?

Perhaps the answer to this is too obvious. He is depressed because he has had a stroke, and it would be most unusual if he were not depressed.

However, let us break it down a bit in order to better understand how the patient feels and the different things which contribute to his depression.

One of the most important causes of depression is fear, and with some people who have had strokes, this fear reaches the proportions of terror. It is fear of what the future holds, fear of what has happened, fear of the unknown. To be most helpful to the patient we must understand the fear and try to dispel it.

Another element of depression is unexpressed anger. The person with a stroke has good cause for anger: he is angry at whatever has caused his stroke—fate, destiny, sometimes God, his work, his family, or anything else he might consider responsible. He is angry and frustrated over his inability to do the things he did before, all the way from the ordinary activities of daily life (walking, dressing, bathing) to going to work; he may be angry that he is changed, different.

Some patients show obvious anger in addition to being depressed. A patient we recall who had severe aphasia was furious with anyone with whom he came in contact, including the doctor. He rarely accepted suggestions for treatment without great protestations, and sometimes he refused treatment outright.

The degree of anger and depression will depend on the patient's basic personality, but everyone with a stroke will experience it.

Another cause of depression is anxiety, which is related to fear. It is different from fear in that it may have no basis in reality. The patient worries about things that really don't require it.

One can say very little that will apply to everyone about how long depression lasts. Recovery is the best antidote, and in those who do not recover completely, time is important. The doctor may prescribe a medication to try and alleviate it, but perhaps the best medicine of all is a warm, loving, understanding family. Above all one must not share the patient's depression or allow one's own fears and worries to join with his.

In some instances this problem is severe enough to require the help of a psychiatrist; the best judge of this is the patient's doctor.

10. Why is the patient more depressed on Saturdays and Sundays?

This is to be expected since there is usually less to do on the weekend and more time to brood about one's misfortune. The patient with a stroke is really no different in this regard from many people without strokes who don't think about their problems while they're at work during the week but tend to become depressed about them on the weekend. It has been observed that many people become depressed over long holidays, perhaps for the same reason.

If the patient is participating in a rehabilitation program, either as an inpatient or an outpatient, he is more likely to show this weekend depression. When he's at the center he is with his disability peers, people like himself. At home he will be among normal people, and the contrast is depressing. Also weekends are often associated with family gatherings, a time for relaxation and fun; the knowledge that these old patterns are now changed may also increase depression.

Finally, home is where he remembers himself as he was before, and the blow to his self-image is more intense there.

11. Why are patients in a better mood when they're busy, receiving therapy, or with friends rather than family?

Keeping busy is a wonderful way to keep one's spirits up, and this applies to a stroke patient as well as to anyone else. It pays to bear it in mind, for the person who has had a stroke may have a lot of time to think about his (or her) troubles. Your ingenuity may be strained to find things he can do. Television is a lifesaver sometimes, but it can be deadly for a person if it is the only diversion. Usually the stroke patient wants to do something himself—the problem is finding the right activity. A rehabilitation center may have the people and projects to help you solve this problem.

In answer to the second part of the question, the various therapies available at a rehabilitation center are wonderful for a patient. They not only provide something to do, but the patient knows that the therapy is contributing to his recovery. It should be no surprise if the patient is happier when he is there working on his rehabilitation.

If the patient is in a better mood with friends, it means that he is being diverted from thinking about himself by his friends or, like so many of us, that he allows himself to be moody when he is at home, but he never does outside of home.

All of the reactions mentioned in this answer apply to most people, disabled or not.

12. Does a patient get depressed when he sees other stroke patients?

The idea that this happens is often a projection of the feelings of the family onto the patient. Interestingly, patients usually are not depressed by associating with other stroke patients. On the contrary they are often cheered by the friendship that results from common misfortune. Further, they are much too preoccupied by their own problems to be distressed by someone else's. It is for these reasons that many rehabilitation centers do not recommend private rooms.

13. Why does the stroke patient cry so easily?

This is an important question because there is a great deal of confusion in the minds of family members about why a patient may cry so easily. One woman said that she and her daughters decided that father now cried easily because he had become "softer and less stern" than he was before the stroke. Others are frightened or very disturbed by it, particularly when the patient is a man. Many think it is a bad sign.

The first thing to be said is that it is practically universal after a stroke. This leads us to believe that some of the damage is located in a part of the brain where the emotions are controlled. That idea is fortified by the fact that the patient will often cry when there seems to be no reason for it. In other words his "cry control center," if there is such a thing, has been temporarily damaged. Many times, of course, the crying is appropriate as when the patient is talking about his stroke or about people who are close to him like children, family, or old friends.

This symptom always disappears, although it may take months or years; there are rare exceptions to this.

14. Why does the patient sometimes laugh inappropriately?

This is the converse of the preceding question, and to some extent the reason is the same—that is, that the portion of the brain which controls emotions may be temporarily impaired. However, just as depression may play a role in crying, there may be other factors in excessive laughter. If the patient's judgment is not good, he may laugh at things which are not particularly funny. Sometimes patients feel the need to deny or hide their feelings of depression and put on a very jovial front. Occasionally they laugh and cry at the same time; in these cases it is likely that there is impairment in the emotion control center.

15. Why does the patient sometimes act childish?

It seems that illnessess of all kinds bring out the child in most of us. Literature is full of stories about big, strong men who become babies when they're sick. This is, of course, exaggerated, but it is perfectly true that the sicker one is, the greater his tendency to be dependent.

At the beginning most stroke patients are actually dependent, for an arm or leg may be without function. But because of the psychological shock of a stroke, the desire to be cared for often persists. Those who live and work with the patient can help alleviate this by gently insisting that he do as much for himself as possible. One must not fall into the trap of retarding the patient's progress by helping him too much.

16. Why are patients sometimes aggressive when they never were before?

The aggressiveness referred to in this question is usually of a mild type such as a slap, a push, or a pinch, but it is indeed a form of violence and is often totally foreign to the patient. At least we think it's foreign to him. In actual fact there are potentialities for violence in all of us. Perhaps that's why we like to read about it in newspapers or novels, see it in the movies or on television; we are dissipating some of our underlying desire to do violence in this fashion. The reason we don't actually do it ("act out" the feeling) is because most of us are in good control of ourselves, and the anger inside is not that great.

Now let us imagine the rage and frustration which the patient with a stroke must feel. Anger often shows itself as depression, which one sees almost universally in stroke patients. But it may manifest itself as anger, too, and be strong enough to cause the patient to hit or scratch. If it is very frequent or very violent, it is something to take up with your doctor since it can be more serious than we have described. Fortunately, serious violence is very rare after a stroke.

17. Why does the patient lose his temper and shout now when he never did before?

There are two possible reasons. Most commonly such behavior results from anger and frustration, the reasons for which have been described. One can hardly expect self-control in the face of a frustrating disability.

If anger is the reason for screaming and shouting, its expression should be allowed. On the other hand good judgment must be used. The family may be sympathetic, but they may discover that ignoring a tantrum will stop it or even that it is necessary to set some kind of limits. Patients require greater consideration than people who are well, but it may not be beneficial to be completely liberal.

Far less frequently, this kind of behavior is the direct result of injury to brain cells and may improve as healing goes on. It is best managed by attempting to calm the patient or by distracting him in some fashion. Sedative drugs are sometimes necessary.

18. Why do stroke patients sometimes get fixed on unimportant things?

In the answers to previous questions in this chapter, it has been pointed out that a stroke may alter a patient's behavior. Although we cannot say precisely why, this tendency to fixation on the unimportant is one of these changes. For example, a patient may insist on being called Kenneth instead of Ken or demand that his wife visit him at exactly 4 P.M. each day and so on. This can be very trying, and family members are often both worried and annoyed by it. One can only suggest patience and fortitude.

19. The patient doesn't seem to be able to concentrate on anything for long. Why not?

This may result from a number of things. In the first few weeks most patients can't concentrate because they are still suffering from the shock of the stroke. As stated earlier, they are upset, frightened, angry, and depressed. In some cases these feelings persist for many months, and concentration may be difficult during that time.

Other patients sustain some damage to the thinking center of the brain, and difficulty concentrating is directly related to this. Fortunately, this can improve, although it may take many months.

Still another cause is the fact that many patients are easily fatigued after a stroke. Doctors cannot yet explain this phenomenon, but it seems that there is a change in the body's general metabolism. This, too, can make concentration difficult.

20. Why does the patient refuse to go out?

This is undoubtedly a result of feelings of shame and loss of self-esteem. The patient does not want to be seen in public or by his friends. He is ashamed of the fact that he is different, changed in some way. Sometimes the problem is relatively small, a minor limp or a slight speech loss, but to the patient it is enough—his image has been tarnished, and he cannot bear to be seen as he is.

The approach to this problem is at the same time simple and difficult. He will resist, but he must be urged to get out among friends. Only by exposure to people will he learn that they still respect and like him for what he is. This works, though it may be very difficult to convince the patient at first.

21. If the patient was considerate before, will he be after a stroke?

Generally yes. A person's basic personality is not permanently changed by a stroke, although this may be hard to believe at the beginning.

We recall the case of a young woman who had a stroke and at times was quite abusive to her children. This woman was angered and frustrated by her stroke to the point where she often lost control and expressed her anger at whoever was around her, including the children. She ceased doing this when she became better able to cope with her problem.

However, it is always a shock to see changes in a person's behavior. If you've lived with someone for thirty or forty years and he suddenly acts differently, it is very frightening. The key to the situation is understanding. Once you know why he does what he does and realize that he is basically the same person, it is possible to feel comfortable with him again.

22. Does the patient know his own limitations?

Most do. As a matter of fact, the majority of stroke patients are very cautious and some actually exaggerate their limitations.

The person who doesn't act this way has probably sustained a very serious stroke or is very old and may have had a similar difficulty before the stroke.

23. How should I treat the patient?

A very important question since it is easy to make mistakes. Let's look at some of the common errors:

1. Because the patient needs so much done for him at the beginning of his illness and because he may have trouble communicating, there is a strong tendency to treat him like a child. This is intensified by the patient's own desire to be taken care of and by the fact that crying comes so easily. It has been pointed out in previous answers that the impairments brought on by a stroke cause feelings of inferiority and shame. Treating someone like a child is bound to increase these feelings and will certainly reinforce the patient's desire to be dependent.

2. Don't treat him like an invalid. After the acute phase of the illness is over, there may be residual impairments. Hopefully, these will disappear, but if they don't the pa-

tient should not be considered sick. Whatever problems remain will not threaten his life nor become worse. They are obstacles to overcome.

3. He is not mentally retarded and should not be so treated. There are details about this in the answer to Question 1. Remember that isolated intellectual impairments do not add up to mental retardation.

4. Don't speak to the patient as though he were deaf. This happens most often if there is a communication problem. We automatically raise our voices if we think we're not being understood. Of course, speaking in a loud voice is no help since there is usually nothing wrong with the patient's hearing. It is not impaired by a stroke because there are centers for hearing on both sides of the brain.

A person may, indeed, be changed by a stroke—temporarily or permanently—but we ought not aggravate his problems by adding disabilities which don't exist.

24. How much should I do for the patient?

This depends upon the stage of his illness. During the first few weeks he will obviously need a great deal of help. However, once he has started the rehabilitation process, at home or in the hospital, one must avoid the tendency to do too much for him. The patient should be encouraged to struggle, and he should be helped only if his task is obviously impossible. Later, when he has become independent, he should be urged to travel or stay at home by himself.

The basic philosophy of rehabilitation is to assist people with a disability to become self-sufficient, for this restores confidence and dignity and makes life worth living again. Few people are so badly disabled that they cannot learn to take care of themselves.

The great majority of stroke patients can and do become self-sufficient. One can either help or hinder this process by the amount of help one gives. It is better to do too little than too much.

25. Should the patient be reprimanded when he is rude to other patients or friends?

We have already discussed the importance of not treating the patient like a child. To reprimand him or speak to him in a condescending fashion will intensify his feelings of inferiority and dependence. Despite the disability, he should bear the responsibility for his own behavior.

26. What does one do if the patient is disinhibited in public?

This is not a very likely possibility, but in some patients it may occur during the first few weeks after a stroke. Naturally one feels embarrassed, but people will usually realize that the patient has been ill and will make allowances.

It is best to be very matter-of-fact in such situations and to ignore the behavior. If it is an outburst of anger, this is the most effective approach, for a show of anger is for the benefit of people in the vicinity. If one doesn't acknowledge it, the anger dies very quickly.

It does little good to try to argue the patient out of his behavior or "discipline" him. He would not act the way he does if he had the capacity to monitor his own behavior. Telling him to do so does no good.

27. Should business problems be discussed with a patient?

Once he has passed the acute phase of his illness we see no reason why almost anything should not be discussed with a patient. Remember that he has had a fearful experience;

his life has been threatened, and he may be left with a disturbing disability. In many patients there is little that will seem important or theatening after such an experience. We frequently observe what the French call *belle indifférence;* the patients just don't get very concerned about things that may have bothered them before.

Remember, too, that it may be beneficial to involve the patient in something important. It diverts his mind from himself, and it may help to restore some of his feelings of self-confidence and reverse his tendency to be dependent.

But this should not be carried too far. If there are business problems which are obviously beyond the patient's competence and are too much for family members, they should promptly seek legal or financial advice. It's surprising how often people will struggle with such matters before looking for help.

28. Should a patient be told bad news, such as the death of a relative?

This question is usually asked because there is concern that bad news may shock the patient and cause him to get worse or have another stroke. In our experience we have not seen this happen. Of course, situations vary and one must use good judgment. In general, patients react in very much the same way as they would have before the stroke. Sometimes they will react very little and at other times be somewhat more emotional, but this is not harmful. Crying is an emotional outlet that is very beneficial, for men as well as for women.

As we have said before, overprotecting the stroke patient does far more harm than good.

29. Should I try to get the patient's mind off himself and onto my troubles?

A good idea, if you can do it without making him anxious.

The patient is naturally very ego centered after a stroke, as with any serious illness. Involving him in the family's problems may serve both to get his mind off himself and to give him a greater feeling of being a normal, participating member of the family. It may be difficult, but every effort should be made to have the patient function as he did before.

We recall a woman who had lost her speech and the use of her right arm. She had been a proud homemaker for years—a wonderful cook and baker, excellent with a needle and thread. She would go home from the rehabilitation center on weekends and sit around watching her daughters do all the things she had done before. She was a very unhappy woman until someone realized that she could still advise and direct her girls in those activities which she had done so well. This seems so obvious but it's surprising how infrequently it's done.

30. Should I encourage the patient by telling him he'll be back at his old job soon?

If the physician believes that it is a good possibility, yes. If you are doing it just to bolster his spirits, no. Reality is often hard to live with, but sooner or later it must be faced.

We do not believe it is wise to say anything about the future in the early weeks after a stroke has occurred. At this point the emphasis should be on getting well and developing self-sufficiency. As time goes on and it becomes clear that the patient will either recover completely or have some residual difficulty, then there can be realistic discussions about the future.

139

31. Why don't our friends come to visit anymore?

Unfortunately, this is a common question, for it is a common problem. One is tempted to become angry and resentful toward friends who fade away, but it is more constructive to try and understand their feelings and do something to prevent this from happening.

It is likely that the most common reason why people stay away is that they're afraid to see anyone changed. This may be due to a strong identification with the patient—a kind of "There, but for the grace of God, go I." Or, it may simply be that the person is very sensitive to misfortune in others.

Whatever the reason, this reaction can be anticipated, and for the sake of the patient, friends should be contacted and reassured. Call them and tell them you know how they may feel, that it is quite natural, and invite them to visit. Your attitude must be matter-of-fact and cheerful, or they will surely be frightened away. We do not mean to imply that this is all very simple, but it is very important that it be done.

This problem is often reinforced by the patient's own reluctance to be with people. It places a great responsibility on the family member. One must be a host or hostess under difficult circumstances, but we have seen it done successfully with immense benefit to the patient.

32. Should I encourage friends and relatives to visit?

By all means. One must resume the normal patterns of living as soon as possible. Though arranging such visits may be difficult at first because of the many reasons which have already been discussed, the knowledge that friends and relatives are interested eventually overcomes the patient's reluctance to see them.

This should not be overdone, since large numbers of visitors are often distressing to the patient, particularly if they all arrive at the same time.

The real problem is that friends may not visit much, and one must try to reestablish normal patterns.

33. What about sexual relationships?

Sexual matters are often neglected in both health and illness. Although we consider our society to be sophisticated and modern, there is a substratum of puritanism which runs deep and wide. This appears to be changing, but it will be a long time before we shall treat the subject of sex with the intelligence and objectivity which it requires.

Although most stroke patients are in the "senior citizen" age group, many are not. Furthermore, a number of studies have revealed that sexual activity often continues in the elderly and is an important part of the life pattern. The matter may, therefore, require discussion.

In our experience one of the questions which is uppermost in the minds of both the patient and his spouse is "Will sexual intercourse bring on another stroke?" One cannot answer this with a categorical "yes" or "no." Strokes are not generally caused by sudden bursts of physical activity, although with a certain type of stroke they sometimes are. This aspect of the problem must therefore be discussed with your physician. Bear in mind, however, that making love may take many forms, and a couple must intelligently explore how best to satisfy their needs for each other. To rule out sexual relationships completely is rarely necessary.

Another concern is that sexual activity may retard the recovery process; there is no evidence we know of that this is so.

It is a fact, however, that many couples will not continue previous patterns after one of them has had a stroke. There must be many reasons: Often they fear further trouble, as stated above; for some it is a relief and an escape from the "responsibility" of a sexual life which they neither enjoyed nor desired prior to the illness; in some cases libido, or the desire for sex, is lost, and it may or may not return. For many male patients it is the practical matter of not being able to maneuver physically as they did before because of weakness of the arm and leg on one side.

If the change in sexual patterns is a problem for either one of a couple, it should be brought up and discussed with a doctor, psychiatrist, or psychologist.

It is an interesting fact that an occasional patient will have an increased desire for sex after a stroke. The explanation for this can be found only in the knowledge of that patient's particular case. It demonstrates, however, that having a stroke is not necessarily associated with changes for the worse in a person's sexual life.

A word about the role of the well partner in this matter. He or she bears a special responsibility in matters of sex and hopefully will be able to assume it. This partner must be willing to change patterns and perhaps assume new roles. Since this is not a textbook on sexual relationships, it is not appropriate to pursue the subject further. We only urge that these matters be explored if they are causes for concern or conflict.

34. Do family relationships change after someone has had a stroke?

This depends entirely on what they were before the stroke.

Whether it's temporary or permanent, a stroke means trouble, and if all was not well among family members before the stroke, it will surely be worse after. A couple who were not getting along may find it even more difficult with all of the tensions and practical problems that a serious illness brings. Adolescent children, already having a difficult time making their transitions, may become more anxious and insecure.

We don't mean to be alarmist, but such things have been observed in many families. It means that one must be realistic and seek professional help if it's necessary. Psychologists and psychiatrists are trained to help people who are having such problems, or one may prefer first to call on his priest, rabbi, or minister for counseling.

But not all relationships are worse after a stroke. Most people are able to meet their new problems and solve them. Some describe very positive changes. This can best be illustrated by the experience of a man whose wife had a very serious stroke. Fortunately he was retired for he now found that he had to be cook, homemaker, and even nurse. He said one day "Although it's difficult, somehow I feel more alive now then I did before and, you know, I took my wife for granted before—I have feelings of affection for her now that I haven't had for thirty years."

A younger man who had a head injury which resulted in symptoms much like a stroke said that he now spent more time with his boy, and that he and his son had grown closer since the accident.

Difficult times often cause people to look at themselves in ways they haven't done before. If any good can be said to come from a stroke, perhaps it is this—that we may stop to look at where we have been and where we are going.

35. People don't realize what the family has to go through when someone has had a stroke. Should there be some consideration for family members?

This is a very important question. Although we realize that the patient is the one who is suffering most, a lot of thought and attention has to be given to members of the family. The occurrence of a stroke usually means that everyone in the family will have to make adjustments, and sometimes they are very great. For example, the husband may have to do things for which he is totally unprepared, like shopping, cooking, and cleaning. A wife may have to begin handling the family finances, go out and get a job, or take over the family business. Children may have new responsibilities or chores. Everyone concerned is usually depressed and frightened about the future. Children sometimes begin to have new problems like failing in school or withdrawing from their usual activities.

It is important that family members be considered not only because they will need help adjusting to their problems, but because they cannot help the patient if they are upset themselves. It is a psychological truism that you cannot do very much for someone else if you're not feeling well yourself. Family members need all the strength they can muster to meet the problems which a stroke often brings, and therefore, they, too, often need help.

36. Is it natural to become impatient or intolerant of someone who has had a stroke?

We mentioned in response to the last question that the reactions and needs of family members are important and should be considered. Sometimes the burdens imposed by such an illness create severe tensions within a family, and one will see evidence of short tempers, impatience, and intolerance. This is simply one more indication of the fact that a stroke usually affects many people. Both the patient and those who are close to him need understanding and a knowledge of what is going on.

We recall a woman who was very impatient with her husband. She thought that he was not doing certain things just to be perverse and stubborn. It took her a while before she understood that no matter how hard he tried he simply could not perform these activities because a particular part of the brain had been temporarily damaged.

We have also said earlier that poor relationships which existed before a stroke may very well get worse afterwards. If a family member finds himself reacting in some negative fashion, it is best to look for professional help, for someone to talk to who can help him to understand himself and the problems he is facing.

37. Should a patient go back to a tense business?

This question is often asked and is one of many which are concerned with the family's attempt to protect the patient.

It is hard to answer categorically. One would want to know how tense the business was, and, even more important, how the patient reacted to the situation after he got back. We are now talking about a person who has recovered enough to be able to go back to work; who can move about almost as well as he did before; and who can talk, read, write, and calculate normally. If the patient reacts to his job the same way he did prior to his stroke, assuming the job made him tense and nervous, then he should be dissuaded from returning. He may be able to work fewer hours or at an easier job. Bear in mind that for some people work is indeed "holy"—that it represents the most important part of their lives. One cannot forbid it without very good reason.

There is another factor involved here which was alluded to before. It is natural for the patient's family and close friends to want to protect him. It is one thing to help the patient whenever he needs it, to give him both physical and moral support. But it will retard his recovery if he is over-protected and overassisted. A stroke patient desperately needs feelings of worth and independence, and one should do nothing to retard the acquisition of these.

38. Do people with strokes need to see a psychiatrist?

Perhaps—but that doesn't mean they are mentally ill. Most of us could well use the help of a psychiatrist many times during the course of our lives.

We believe that one of the basic troubles in the world is that there are too many people who don't understand themselves, who don't understand why they do what they do and say what they say. Learning about oneself is probably the most important bit of education any one of us can get, and yet, paradoxically, it is the most neglected part of people's education.

The person who has had a stroke (and his family) are subjected by that misfortune to a tremendous strain. It is most important that they find help in meeting those stresses, and a psychiatrist may be needed to provide it.

CHAPTER 5

Rehabilitation

1. What does rehabilitation really mean; what does it include?
2. When does rehabilitation begin?
3. How soon can the patient be out of bed?
4. Should the patient be taught to walk while he's in the general hospital?
5. Should the patient's blood pressure be checked every day?
6. Should "blood thinners" be used after a stroke?
7. What medications are helpful for the stroke patient?
8. Can surgery help cure a stroke?
9. Will hypnosis help a stroke patient?
10. What else can be done in the hospital in the early weeks after a stroke?
11. Why do the hand and ankle swell?
12. What specific joints are liable to become deformed and how is this prevented?
13. What can be done about spasticity?
14. When is the patient ready for intensive rehabilitation?
15. Where can one get rehabilitation after a stroke?
16. Does a patient need a special duty nurse when he is first admitted to a rehabilitation center?

17. Who makes up the rehabilitation team one hears so much about?
18. What is a doctor called who is a specialist in rehabilitation medicine?
19. Is there such a thing as a rehabilitation nurse?
20. What is a physical therapist and what does he do for the stroke patient?
21. Does physical therapy bring about return of function?
22. Does physical therapy increase the skill and endurance of the hemiplegic arm and leg as in the training of an athlete?
23. What is an orthotist?
24. What is a brace, when is it necessary, and who makes it?
25. What are slings and splints and when are they used?
26. What is an occupational therapist and what does the patient do in occupational therapy?
27. What is taught in the way of homemaking? Are there visits to the home?
28. What is the role of the social worker in stroke rehabilitation?
29. What does the psychologist do in the rehabilitation of the stroke patient?
30. What is a vocational counselor and what does he do for the stroke patient?
31. What is a recreation therapist?
32. What do volunteer workers do in a rehabilitation program?
33. What is a typical treatment program and how is it planned?
34. What is the usual course of a stroke patient who is admitted for rehabilitation and how long does it take?
35. Must one be content if the patient can only walk with a brace and cane?

36. Why are some patients able to walk at the rehabilitation center but not at home on weekends?
37. When should a patient be treated as an inpatient and when as an outpatient?
38. How long should the patient be in rehabilitation treatment?
39. Can a stroke patient be treated at home?
40. Should someone who has had a stroke drive a car?
41. Can a patient take an air trip? What are the effects of high altitude?
42. Where can I get help?

Introduction

The concept of medical rehabilitation is, of necessity, very broad. In a sense all of medicine is rehabilitation because the purpose of the healing arts is to return the patient to normal living, but it remained for a few pioneers, chief among them Dr. Howard A. Rusk, founder of the Institute of Rehabilitation Medicine in New York, to make both the medical and nonmedical world aware of the needs of people with chronic illness. To these patients rehabilitation has a very special meaning, for it opens doors that society had previously believed to be irrevocably locked.

Those who practice rehabilitation medicine are not purveyors of magic or miracles. They deal in concern for the human being who has sustained a severe illness, concern for every aspect of his existence. Their tools are the tools of traditional medicine and the skills of doctors and a host of other professionals whose special knowledge can be turned to the patient's benefit. Above all, they believe in the dignity of the individual, regardless of his infirmities. Rehabilitation is a struggle against the indignity of illness in some of its most difficult forms. As a medical specialty it is young, but the ethical principles upon which it is based are as old as civilization.

It would not be appropriate to describe the rehabilitation process in great detail in this book. However, we shall try to indicate how the problems of the stroke patient are approached, what can be expected, and what is beyond the scope of rehabilitation medicine.

1. What does rehabilitation really mean; what does it include?

Rehabilitation after stroke means helping the patient to use fully whatever remaining capacities he has. In some cases this means learning to do things with one hand that he did before with two, or walking with a brace. Whatever the details, the goal of rehabilitation is to help every patient resume his life as it was before, regardless of disability.

As we said in Chapter 4, it is hard for a person to adjust to the fact that physically he is not what he was before. Since getting old is a gradual process, we have time to adjust to it, but a stroke happens suddenly. In a moment a person may be changed rather radically.

Difficult though it may be, isn't this the same adjustment which all must make with advancing age—only faster? As we work with the patient and teach him the many things there are to learn in a rehabilitation program, we try to help him make this adjustment, for in a sense adjusting is the major problem. The patient must learn to cope with his changed condition, to realize that there are values more important than how well one walks or moves an arm. Of course, these are important, but if one is faced with irrevocable change, he must try to grow in the mind and substitute the pleasures and joys of the mind for physical ones.

The rehabilitation process is many things—*physical therapy* to help the patient use his limbs better, walk better; *occupational therapy* to increase function through special methods; *speech pathology* to identify and help the patient overcome a speech problem; *psychology and psychiatry* to explore the mental and emotional faculties of the patient; *social service* to assist in the solution of home and community problems; *vocational counseling* to explore returning to work; *orthotics* to provide braces and splints so that the patient can use his arms and legs better; *therapeutic recreation,* which is exactly what it sounds like; all the traditional diagnostic facilities of a hospital and the special one of electrodiagnosis which is used so much in rehabilitation; and, as in every field of medicine, the nurse and the doctor.

We shall go into more detail on the role of each of these professional disciplines in the process of rehabilitation for the person with a stroke.

Having mentioned the members of the rehabilitation team, it must be emphasized that rehabilitation is a concept which can be practiced where there is no team. For example, there are small communities that do not have physical, occupational, and speech therapists. Nurses are often called upon to learn the techniques of rehabilitation, and along with practical nurses and aides, they do a splendid job. They cannot be all things to all people, but when the situation demands it, nurses are ideally suited to substitute for their colleagues from other therapies.

For the most thorough job of rehabilitation, it should be the goal of every community to assemble a rehabilitation team.

2. When does rehabilitation begin?

In a real sense rehabilitation begins the moment after someone has sustained a stroke. The reason is clear if one considers the goals of rehabilitation: to prevent unnecessary disability resulting from neglect or insufficient treatment; to evaluate the capacities of an individual after a serious illness; to help the patient utilize his residual capacities to the full, using all the tools of medicine and nonmedical science which are available. To put it more plainly, we try to prevent complications, find out what the person can do, and then teach him to do those things so that he can return to a way of life as similar as possible to the one he lived before.

When we talk of preventing complications, we mean specifically such things as "freezing" of the joints which can prevent normal movement, deformities due to joint "freezing," weakness resulting from disuse rather than from the illness itself. These are the most important complications after a stroke, aside from those involving the internal organs.

As we go through this chapter there will be frequent mention of the rehabilitation team. This refers to the various professionals who participate in the rehabilitation process. Aside from the doctor, the first member of this team to contact the patient is the nurse. Her role can be crucial since she sees the patient when he is at his sickest and most helpless—at the beginning. A joint can stiffen in a very short time while the patient is bedridden, but if the body part is kept in a good position by the appropriate use of pillows, sandbags, wooden boards, etc., a permanent *contracture* can be avoided. Proper positioning plus moving the limb a few times a day obviates this complication.

For example, the foot tends to fall when a leg is paralyzed, and if left untended, the heel cord will shorten and the foot will be fixed in a position with the toe pointed. The nurse who is trained in these matters arranges the patient in bed so that the foot is kept at a 90-degree angle with the leg. In addition, she moves the foot through its full range of motion a few times each day. The importance of this kind of care can't be overestimated. In an advanced center where there is a staff of physical therapists, some of these procedures are carried out by them, but it is valuable for the nurse to perform these functions too since she is with the patient so much of the time. Furthermore, many hospitals do not have a physical therapist, and the responsibility falls entirely to the nurse.

At this point a well-trained nurse contributes in another

way. Again, because of her intimate contact with the patient and family, she can explain some of the things which are happening, why certain procedures are being done, and so forth. Of course, some questions are discussed with the doctor, but there are many that the nurse can answer. A well-trained, sensitive nurse knows what a frightening, difficult time it is for the patient and his family, and she can be a great source of comfort and support.

Rehabilitation begins with the prevention of physical complications and that begins immediately.

3. How soon can the patient be out of bed?

This is a decision which the attending physician will make, and it depends on such things as the degree of alertness of the patient, whether his heart and blood pressure are stable, whether the process which caused the stroke is complete, whether the patient has sufficient energy to sit up.

This is the first step—to sit on the edge of the bed with support and dangle the legs. He then graduates to standing for a few moments, always with support, and then perhaps to taking a few steps to a nearby chair.

Sometimes this process can be started a few days after the stroke. Everyone now appreciates that prolonged bed rest is not good unless it is absolutely necessary.

4. Should the patient be taught to walk while he's in the general hospital?

If his condition has stabilized as described in the preceding answer, and if there is a trained therapist available, there is no reason why he should not begin walking training. Ordinarily general hospitals are anxious to discharge patients once they have stabilized because of the need for beds; thus, the rehabilitation process must be carried on elsewhere or with the patient as an outpatient. Some general hospitals have rehabilitation services where patients are transferred from medicine or neurology to continue their training. There is great variation, and all depends upon the condition of the patient and the trained medical people and facilities available in the hospital.

5. Should the patient's blood pressure be checked every day?

This is entirely an individual matter and depends on whether he has a history of high blood pressure, is taking medications which are liable to cause the pressure to go up or down, whether he has heart trouble, and many other such factors.

The attending physician will decide on such matters and write appropriate orders when the patient is admitted.

6. Should "blood thinners" be used after a stroke?

Anticoagulants, as they are known, are used by some physicians after a stroke to prevent a recurrence. However, it should be pointed out immediately that the decision to use them or not is based upon many considerations which the doctor must evaluate. There is evidence that certain patients do just as well without them.

The principle behind the use of these drugs and how they were discovered is a very interesting chapter in medical history. It came about through the study of a bleeding disease in cows. It was found that these cows developed a tendency to bleed after eating spoiled sweet clover and that the substance in the clover which was responsible was something called "dicoumarin." Blood-thinning drugs commonly in use today are derived directly from this substance. By interfering with the body's blood clotting mechanism in a controlled fashion, anticoagulants are able to prevent clot formation in some cases.

Scientists continue to work on all aspects of the stroke

problem, and it may very well be that today's research will bring forth new methods of treatment that are valuable and applicable to all cases of stroke.

7. What medications are helpful for the stroke patient?

There are no medications which are specific for stroke: that is, those medications which are employed for stroke patients are also used in many other conditions.

For example, tranquilizers are sometimes very helpful, but as everyone knows they are used in a wide variety of conditions. They are indicated for the patient who is very anxious or excitable.

Perhaps of even greater importance are the so-called anti-depressant drugs since so many stroke patients are depressed. These drugs are not surefire, but they are often very helpful.

Another group of drugs are those prescribed in an attempt to relieve spasticity. Unfortunately, they are not as effective as might be desired, but sometimes they can modify this unpleasant symptom. Most of these drugs are related to tranquilizers.

In certain situations anticoagulant drugs (blood thinners) are used after a stroke. They are most commonly used to prevent stroke, as we indicated in the previous answer: The attending doctor will know whether or not to employ them.

Since many stroke patients are in the older age group, they often require heart or blood pressure medication and other medications in this category. One cannot possibly give an exhaustive list of all of these.

8. Can surgery help cure a stroke?

Unfortunately there is as yet no therapeutic surgical procedure which will do what preventive surgery does. In the latter case, if the narrowing in the blood vessel is in an artery in the neck or chest, there is a possibility of doing something about it before it causes a stroke. This was discussed more fully in Question 22, Chapter 1.

The problem with a completed stroke is that the damage is done in the first few minutes; it is common knowledge that brain tissue cannot do without oxygen for more than ten minutes at the most. There are situations in which quick surgery is important, but these are relatively rare and have to do with hemorrhage. Most strokes are not caused by hemorrhage and cannot be helped by surgery.

9. Will hypnosis help a stroke patient?

The person who asks this question usually means "Will hypnosis help get rid of the weakness of the arm or leg or the speech problem if there is one?"—and the answer is that it will not. The reason is that the trouble in stroke is due to damage of brain tissue, and hypnosis has no effect on this. If someone has a broken arm, it cannot be mended by hypnotism. Similarly the results of a stroke cannot be changed by hypnosis.

10. What else can be done in the hospital in the early weeks after a stroke?

This depends upon where the patient is and the training of the hospital personnel. In some cases well-trained nurses can and must carry on the process of early rehabilitation under medical direction. In others there are physical and occupational therapists to do the job, alone or with the nursing staff.

Let us assume the patient is in a general hospital, and it is the period immediately following the stroke. Once he has begun to move about, he can be taught a number of things. Turning in bed, for example, seems like a simple thing, but it must be taught to many patients. Getting out of bed may be even more difficult. Learning how to get in and out of a wheelchair, from the wheelchair to an easy chair or the toilet, may also be taught at this stage.

Occupational therapists engaged in rehabilitation have traditionally been concerned with activities requiring the skilled use of the hands. There will be more detail about this later. It is mentioned here to indicate that, depending upon the setting, such things as teaching the patient to shave, comb his hair, and feed himself can be started in the general hospital, either by an occupational therapist or a nurse. Often nurses are the only professionals available for some of these things, and a good nurse can be exceedingly important during the early days.

11. Why do the hand and ankle swell?

There are two things which will cause a limb to swell, whether it is normal or not. (People who take long airplane trips often find their feet swollen upon arriving at their destinations.) These two things are *immobility* and the so-called *dependent position*. The latter means that the limb hangs down (either the arm or leg). If a limb remains in this position for a long time, the blood has a hard time returning to the heart. Immobility results in the same thing since muscles in the arm and leg tend to act as a pump. When the muscles contract, they squeeze the veins in and around them, and this helps to push the blood back to the heart. This is not to imply that blood will not get back to the heart in a stroke patient or that it is a dangerous situation. What it means is that the blood will be slower in getting back, and this allows water to leak out of the blood vessels and into the tissues. This is the swelling that is seen.

The obvious remedy for this situation is not to allow the limb to hang down for long periods of time and to move it. For the arm, this usually means wearing a sling and exercising it as often as possible. In the leg, it means walking and moving the leg about when the patient is seated. Going to bed at night is a sure cure—the swollen limb is always better in the morning.

Another reason for a swollen hand is the shoulder–hand syndrome which is discussed in Question 25, Chapter 2.

The doctor will always give careful consideration to such problems for there are other reasons for swelling which require other kinds of treatment.

12. What specific joints are liable to become deformed and how is this prevented?

This is the order of frequency in which joint deformities are seen after a stroke: (1) wrist and hand, (2) shoulder, (3) ankle, and (4) knee.

As mentioned elsewhere, joint deformities can almost always be prevented by exercising the involved limbs a few times each day and never allowing the arm or leg to be in a poor position for long periods of time.

One reason why the arm is more susceptible is that it is usually weaker and more spastic than the leg. However, if the leg is kept tightly covered in bed with the foot pushed out straight, the heel cord can shorten, and it will no longer be possible to bend the foot upward. This position of the foot can make walking very difficult.

Taking them in order again, here's what can happen to these joints if they are neglected.

1. *Wrist and hand.* These will be bent, and, if unexercised, will remain in that position. Less often the fingers stiffen in the straightened position.

2. *Shoulder.* If this joint stiffens the patient will not be able to raise his arm forward or to the side. In addition, if the patient doesn't wear a sling in the early stages, there may be stretching of the joint envelope with partial dislocation of the arm from the shoulder socket.

3. *Ankle.* Usually the heel cord will shorten and the foot will not be able to bend upward.

4. *Knee.* This is least common, but, in neglected patients, the knee may be permanently bent.

Occasionally joint deformities are unavoidable. In the great majority of cases proper positioning and frequent moving of the patient in bed as well as daily exercise will prevent these complications. In addition, the patient can be taught to exercise his weak limbs himself. Sometimes splints are prescribed to maintain the hand and wrist in the proper position.

13. What can be done about spasticity?

The nature of spasticity is discussed in Question 13, Chapter 2. It is the "stiffness" which may develop in a stroke patient's arm or leg along with weakness. In the first days and weeks after the stroke, the weak or paralyzed limb is loose, like that of a rag doll. Gradually this turns into stiffness, and it is difficult to bend or straighten the limb, even if this is done by someone for the patient. As recovery goes on to completion this gradually disappears, and the limb once more has the normal degree of looseness when it is moved or bent. If complete recovery does not take place, the limb may remain abnormally stiff. If it is an arm it is carried in the bent position most of the time.

Unfortunately, there is no good method for treating spasticity. There are a few drugs in the tranquilizer family which seem to reduce spasticity a little, but the ideal drug has not yet been found.

Depending on its location and importance, the nerve to a spastic muscle is sometimes cut. This also renders the muscle useless, so this procedure can only be done on muscles which are not important.

More recently there has been an attempt to reduce spasticity by injecting a chemical around the nerve that leads to a spastic muscle. This may diminish the spasticity without causing the patient to lose much strength in the muscle. This is not a completely proved technique but may turn out to be very beneficial.

One very practical though temporary way of relieving this symptom is to work the spastic muscle very hard. This seems to have a good effect for a while, but the spasticity always returns. However, if the exercise is repeated periodically throughout the day, spasticity can be kept less severe.

14. When is the patient ready for intensive rehabilitation?

As soon as he has stabilized. What we mean in medicine by stabilized is that his blood pressure and heart rate are steady, he is able to be up without being weak or dizzy, he has control over elimination functions, he is not confused or disoriented, and he is able to stand for short periods of time, whether or not he can take some steps. The patient may reach this point a few days after a stroke or weeks later. It is rarely a clear-cut time, and one must observe him carefully to determine when to go ahead with the next phase of rehabilitation.

15. Where can one get rehabilitation after a stroke?

There is a mistaken notion that it is necessary to go to a rehabilitation center for this kind of treatment. Of course, such centers usually have the most complete programs because they are exclusively engaged in this kind of work. However, there are departments of rehabilitation medicine or physical medicine in most large hospitals these days, staffed by therapists of various kinds and under the direction of a doctor trained in physical medicine and rehabilitation. Almost all Veterans Administration hospitals have rehabilitation services.

In the answer to Question 42 in this chapter and in the Appendix, suggestions are made as to where one can find help.

The thing to remember is that the rehabilitation of stroke patients requires only knowledge and trained professionals—it does not require elaborate equipment or buildings. Special devices, like leg braces, are often needed, but the doctor will know how to prescribe and secure these. Even in large rehabilitation centers these devices are often made outside of the hospital by private companies.

We shall go into greater detail about all of this in the answers to subsequent questions.

16. Does a patient need a special duty nurse when he is first admitted to a rehabilitation center?

It is difficult to generalize in answering this question, but most patients in a rehabilitation center are well enough not to need a special nurse. One thinks of special nurses as being required when a patient is bedridden. In a rehabilitation center it is usually better for the patient to try and care for himself. Furthermore, there is always a feeling of camaraderie among patients, and they help each other a great deal. The regular nursing staff is capable of providing for all of the patient's nursing needs.

17. Who makes up the rehabilitation team one hears so much about?

Since rehabilitation may involve physical, emotional, social, vocational, and educational aspects of the patient's life, many different kinds of professionals are on this team. We shall describe how each of them participate in the rehabilitation process in the answers that follow.

It is called a "team" because these professionals work together, exchange information about the patient, and, under the leadership of the doctor, make the decisions that are necessary for an effective treatment program. No doubt the composition of this team will change as time goes on, since everything changes with new knowledge and methods.

18. What is a doctor called who is a specialist in rehabilitation medicine?

The name of the specialty is physical medicine and rehabilitation, and the doctor is called a *physiatrist*. This is sometimes confusing to people since the word is so much like *psychiatrist*.

Physiatrists take special training just as surgeons, pediatricians, neurologists, and other specialists do. Upon completion of training, they take examinations; when they pass, they are certified as specialists in this field.

Doctors in this work are trained to understand the many conditions which may result in physical or mental disability and what can be done to help the patient fully utilize his talents and abilities. The physiatrist is the leader of the rehabilitation team and must coordinate the contribution of each of its members. He cannot function without his colleagues in the various disciplines and must see to it that the knowledge of the team members is turned to the patient's benefit. In the final analysis, as in all of medicine, the doctor bears the ultimate responsibility for the patient.

Physiatrists work in rehabilitation centers, general hospitals, nursing homes, industry, government agencies, and private practice.

19. Is there such a thing as a rehabilitation nurse?

There is indeed, and, as stated earlier, the nurse plays a vital role in the treatment of stroke. She may be the only one working with the patient in some circumstances.

Rehabilitation nursing refers to a specific specialty in

nursing, and those who are trained in this field are usually found in rehabilitation centers or large general hospitals. Just as the operating room nurse or the public health nurse are specialists in particular fields, rehabilitation nurses are trained to work with the kinds of patients who come to a rehabilitation center, including those with stroke. They understand the necessity for proper positioning of body parts, care of the skin in paralyzed patients, techniques for teaching the patient to care for himself, and many other details that are important to the stroke patient. All of this is in addition to their usual duties in caring for hospitalized patients.

Rehabilitation nursing, therefore, requires special knowledge of the diseases and conditions which their patients have—in this case, stroke. The nurse is often questioned by both patient and family about the meaning of symptoms and must be knowledgeable so that she can educate and reassure.

She is a member of the rehabilitation team and participates in conferences and decision making. By virtue of her close contact with the patient, she sometimes has information that no one else has.

Nursing is one of the oldest of the medical professions, and everyone recognizes its importance. Today's nurse is more than a doctor's assistant. She is a professional who makes a contribution to the patient's recovery on her own, by virtue of her own knowledge and understanding.

20. What is a physical therapist and what does he do for the stroke patient?

Physical therapists are university-trained, licensed professionals whose specialty is the motor or muscle system of the body. Through their course of study they learn the anatomy and function of the muscles and joints as well as how to apply various methods of treatment. Physical therapists work under the direction of physicians.

When a stroke patient begins a course of rehabilitation

therapy he undergoes various evaluations, one of which is a measurement of the range of motion of the joints and the strength of his muscles. This is performed by physical therapists. In addition they evaluate the patient's ability to care for his daily needs—transfer himself, stand, sit, and walk—the so-called activities of daily living.

Once evaluations have been completed, the physical therapist participates with the rest of the rehabilitation team to design and carry out a program of therapy. The physical therapist works to increase the range of motion of affected joints and to increase the power of the muscles. He does this through exercise and various forms of heat, cold, massage, and careful manipulation. He also may teach the patient those activities of daily living in which he is deficient.

When assistive devices such as braces, splints, slings, special shoes, etc., are required, it is the physical therapist who usually instructs the patients in their proper use.

It is sometimes necessary for a member of the rehabilitation team to visit the patient's home prior to discharge and make recommendations for necessary changes in furniture arrangement, structure, and so forth. Physical therapists, among others, perform this important function.

Finally, they are usually asked to prepare a program of exercises which the patient can use at home after discharge in order to maintain whatever he has achieved through physical therapy treatment.

21. Does physical therapy bring about return of function?

Strictly speaking physical therapy does not cause muscles to regain their normal strength and coordination. That is dependent upon the healing process in the brain. What it does do is make sure that the patient is using all of the power which he does have; it teaches him to use once more muscles which he may have "forgotten" how to use as a result of the stroke; it prevents complications like stiff joints and weakness from lack of use.

This is a very important distinction because patients and their families often believe that it is the therapy which is bringing about the return of function, and that if treatment is continued indefinitely complete recovery will occur. Unfortunately, this is not the case.

It should be mentioned that there are a few clinics in the United States where this idea is taught; that is, that therapy will force the return of function. Fortunately, there are not many of them for this concept is totally without scientific validity. These people have put forth a theory without any evidence that it is true and, in essence, are taking advantage of patients who are anxious to find a cure.

There is no one in medicine who does not wish that it were possible to restore full function to every patient. If continued, intensive therapy were the answer, this would be the prescription for every stroke patient. Patient and family must trust the judgment of the doctor as to when to start and when to stop treatment.

22. Does physical therapy increase the skill and endurance of the hemiplegic arm and leg as in the training of an athlete?

It will certainly increase the endurance of involved limbs, but the matter of skill is dependent on the proper connections between the brain and the arm or leg. While these are disturbed as a result of a stroke, it is not possible for the patient to develop skill or increase coordination. However, as the brain heals and connections are restored, the patient may begin to use the limbs more skillfully and therapy will help this process.

We recall a patient who did not recover normal use of his arm or leg. Despite this he learned to swim almost as well as he had before by dint of hard work and perseverance.

23. What is an orthotist?

This is a question which might even be asked by doctors not associated with rehabilitation, for the term is relatively new and only those in medicine who are in the position of prescribing leg braces or special devices for the hand and arm would encounter an orthotist.

Orthotists are trained professionals who specialize in making braces, splints, and special devices. For example, there are some stroke patients who need a leg brace in order to begin walking; without it the knee might buckle and the ankle would be very unstable. The doctor writes a prescription for the brace specifying exactly what he wants. If he has a particularly difficult problem he may ask the orthotist to discuss it with him since the well-trained orthotist is aware of all the varieties and modifications of braces.

At advanced rehabilitation centers there are orthotists who do research on better methods for bracing. In the past few years some very interesting new designs have emerged from these laboratories.

Although most stroke patients do not require it, the orthotist may be called upon to make a special splint for the hand. These are made from metal, plastic, or plaster and are designed to keep the hand in a normal position or assist in movement of the fingers.

The arm slings which are often prescribed for patients in the early weeks after the stroke may also be made in the orthotist's laboratory.

24. What is a brace, when is it necessary, and who makes it?

The basic concept of bracing for stroke is simple. When as a result of weakness there is instability at the ankle or knee, a brace is employed to prevent collapse or undesirable movement of these joints. Muscles are attached around joints, and when they contract there is movement. If the muscles are weak or paralyzed, movement is reduced or impossible. One cannot stand on such a leg—an attempt to do so results in collapse.

Braces traditionally have been made of metal bars which attach to the shoe and are strapped to the leg. A short leg brace stops below the knee; a long leg brace extends to the upper part of the thigh.

One uses a *short leg brace* if the ankle is weak in order to prevent the front of the foot from dropping down. If it is allowed to drop, the patient trips. This brace also prevents turning of the ankle, which may be a big problem for the stroke patient. Short leg braces are prescribed more than any other kind for stroke patients since the ankle is frequently weak while the knee and hip are strong enough to work on their own.

If a patient's knee buckles when he first begins to walk it means he needs a *long leg brace*. Again, it is attached to his shoe but now extends above the knee. The brace has a joint at the knee for later use but at the beginning it is kept locked. This permits the patient to get up and walk earlier than he ordinarily would, which is good for him psychologically. It also helps him to learn to balance himself and practice walking even though the knee is straight. When he has gained sufficient strength in the proper muscles, the brace is converted to a short leg brace.

If the patient develops enough strength in his ankle muscles, he can discard the short leg brace as well. It is unwise to do this, however, unless sufficient strength has returned. Often this takes many months.

Braces are made by *orthotists*. These are people who are trained in the art of designing, measuring, fitting, and fabricating braces and splints for people with many different kinds of disabilities. They are becoming more and more important in rehabilitation since they are developing new types of braces—ones that look better, do the job better, and sometimes are easier to make. Orthotists often make valuable suggestions to physicians about the best type of brace to use in unusual situations.

25. What are slings and splints and when are they used?

A sling is very commonly used with a stroke patient to prevent the arm from loosening in the shoulder socket. It also keeps the forearm and hand elevated so that swelling will not occur. A sling is very important in the early days after a stroke since this is the time when the arm is liable to be very weak and when it most requires support.

Splints are made of metal, plaster, or plastic. They are used to prevent deformities in the hand and wrist when there is a lot of spasticity. In such cases exercise is not enough to prevent deformity.

26. What is an occupational therapist and what does the patient do in occupational therapy?

This university-trained professional is also devoted to the return of function in disabled limbs as well as the acquisition of skills which make it possible for a patient to live independently. But the occupational therapist approaches the problem in a different way from the physical therapist: the occupational therapist uses actual tasks to increase the coordination and strength of an impaired arm or leg. For example, to strengthen an arm he might choose sanding wood or working a handloom.

The occupational therapist also works with the patient who needs to learn specific activities like dressing, grooming, or eating. If an arm is disabled, this may entail teaching him how these things can be done with only one hand.

169

Certain special responsibilities also fall to the occupational therapist. One of these is the training of women (and occasionally men) in a variety of homemaking activities such as cooking, sewing, and housekeeping. This usually involves energy-saving techniques and the use of special appliances and equipment. Often the therapist goes into the home and recommends architectural or equipment changes, usually in the kitchen.

A very important function of occupational therapy is to conduct what are called prevocational evaluations. In these, the patient is tested in many different kinds of work in order to judge what might be a suitable vocation for him. In this case, vocational counselor and occupational therapist work closely together.

Besides these very practical and important aspects of the rehabilitation process, the occupational therapist also teaches skills which a patient may use in his leisure time, something not to be underestimated in its value.

As with all of the other disciplines, occupational therapists participate in team deliberations and contribute their observations and suggestions.

Many people think that occupational therapists have something to do with helping the patient choose a new occupation or relearn his old one. This is not true. Occupational therapists assist in this process by doing prevocational testing, but the vocational counselor is the one who takes the major responsibility for getting the patient back to work.

27. What is taught in the way of homemaking? Are there visits to the home?

One of the services offered at a rehabilitation center is homemaking training. A large part of this has to do with kitchen activities and involves such things as teaching the patient to use special kitchen utensils and to work from a wheelchair, a high stool, a rolling chair, or while using crutches. Some patients have to learn how to work with one hand; others have visual difficulties that must be taken into account.

After evaluating the patient, the staff member decides what equipment and what approach will be used and starts the training.

Occasionally it is necessary to visit the home in order to see what changes need to be made; such changes may include lowering cupboards, changing methods of storage, widening doorways, and many others.

For the most part women take this training. Occasionally it is necessary for a man to do it if circumstances require his wife to go out to work while he remains at home. It is a reversal of roles that is usually difficult for both husband and wife to accept.

28. What is the role of the social worker in stroke rehabilitation?

The social worker is one of the patient's important links to the outside world; he is trained to assist, advise, and investigate for the patient matters that have to do with home and community. Social work is one of the oldest and most respected professions, and the very nature of rehabilitation problems demands the talents of these professionals.

A stroke often causes problems in the home that may range from the need for special help or equipment to conflicts among family members. Finances are frequently a source of great concern. By getting to know the patient, his family, and his situation and by knowing the sources of help in the community, the social worker contributes valuable information for the many decisions which must be made.

Sometimes he is the best one to counsel the family and to be a continuing source of support during the rehabilitation

171

process. Patients and their families need a knowledgeable, sympathetic ear, and it is one of the cornerstones of training in social work to provide this. Over the years, social workers have become more and more concerned with the psychological trauma of illness to both patient and family, and they are trained to be helpful in this area.

29. What does the psychologist do in the rehabilitation of the stroke patient?

The psychologist is the member of the rehabilitation team whose primary interest is evaluating the patient's intellectual and emotional status. Chapter 4 is devoted to this subject and should provide an idea of the importance and complexity of this part of the stroke problem.

In order to arrive at his conclusions, the psychologist chooses from a large number of tests which he has learned to administer and interpret during his training. These tests measure intelligence, memory of all kinds, perceptual ability, knowledge, reasoning, and so forth. The psychologist is also trained to evaluate the person's judgment, ability to think in abstract terms, and emotional state.

It is important for both patient and family to realize that this is a vital part of the overall evaluation, that all patients are tested psychologically, and that such testing is not done because the patient is thought to be "mental." Some patients resent these tests because they do not understand why they are being done.

Psychologists are also trained to counsel patients and sometimes the family as well. As has been said before, having a stroke and being left with some residual disability is always a severe blow to the patient and family, and they frequently need help adjusting to the situation. In the final analysis, how the patient reacts to his disability is more important than the disability itself. Remember that there are many unhappy, depressed people who have not had strokes and who often need the help of a psychologist or psychiatrist. Little wonder that stroke patients might need such assistance.

Most large psychology departments have one or more members of the staff who do research on the intellectual and emotional problems of stroke. By learning more about the condition, we become better able to treat the patient with new methods or modifications of old ones.

30. What is a vocational counselor and what does he do for the stroke patient?

The vocational counselor is a member of the rehabilitation team with special knowledge of disability as it relates to the world of work. He works closely with other members of the rehabilitation team involved in the treatment of stroke patients and utilizes pertinent information to determine vocational potential. He must take into account all aspects of the patient's physical, mental, emotional, and social condition.

Many patients in the older age group do not require the services of a vocational counselor. They are either retired or about to retire. What follows describes the vocational counselor's role in rehabilitating patients who can return to work.

He has many tasks; an early one is the screening of patients who are eligible for services from the State Division of Vocational Rehabilitation. This agency, which incidentally employs large numbers of vocational counselors, provides counseling service as well as funds to treat, evaluate, and train patients who have work potential.

The main job of the vocational counselor is to try and gauge the stroke patient's vocational ability. This is done by studying his educational and work history and his physical limitations, by testing, and by providing actual work trials or on-the-job evaluations.

All of this may be difficult with the stroke patient, especially if he is one who has aphasia or is not yet ready to think about working. For this reason, counseling sessions are almost routine. The counselor encourages the patient to express his feelings about a vocation, his frustrations, and his fears. The patient is always encouraged to assume responsibility in the process of looking for a new vocation, if a new one is necessary.

Upon completion of the vocational evaluation, the patient may be referred for further training or he may be ready to take a job or work in a sheltered workshop.

Often the responsibility for actual job placement falls to the vocational counselor. This requires liaison with business and industry, educating prospective employers, and instructing patients on how to get and hold a job. The counselor may help the patient in other ways by solving transportation problems, securing adaptive devices, and so forth.

Finally, the vocational counselor follows the patient's progress and remains available for future help and consultation.

31. What is a recreation therapist?

The job of the recreation therapist is easy to imagine but not easy to carry out. He or she designs things for the patient to do in his free time which will both divert him and contribute to overall rehabilitation goals.

It has been repeated many times in this book that the stroke patient who has been left with some disability has tremendous difficulty adjusting to that disability. The reasons for this are discussed in Chapter 4.

One of the commonest problems is that he doesn't like to get out among people for he now feels inferior and unworthy. It is one of the recreation therapist's jobs to combat this tendency and help him realize that being with people is not so frightening and uncomfortable. The proper use of leisure hours is even more important for people who are recovering from a serious illness than it is for those who are well.

174

32. What do volunteer workers do in a rehabilitation program?

In every hospital and rehabilitation center, volunteer workers (usually ladies) do many things to make patients' lives more pleasant. Anyone who has visited or been a patient in a hospital is aware of this.

At the New York University Institute of Rehabilitation Medicine there is a group of volunteers engaged in a pioneer project. It is known as continued therapy, and many stroke patients are participants. Although this activity is not confined to outpatients, the group is largely composed of those who no longer need to be hospitalized.

The concept is straightforward: that many patients need the opportunity to meet together in a comfortable, familiar setting, and that they need continuing physical, conversational, and social stimulation. This program is organized and carried out by trained volunteers, and it has demonstrated its value over the years. If one remembers the great problem that stroke patients have being with people and regaining feelings of confidence and worth, it is not surprising that they derive great benefit from a program like this.

33. What is a typical treatment program and how is it planned?

When a stroke patient is admitted to a rehabilitation center or service, he is examined, his history is taken, and the necessary X-rays and blood tests are done—much the same procedure as with any patient admitted to a hospital. The purpose of this procedure is to identify the nature of his condition so that proper treatment can be instituted.

In a rehabilitation center there are additional tests done. These are called evaluations and are performed by the various members of the team, as previously described. When all

175

of these evaluations are done, the staff meets and, under the direction of the doctor, decides on a program. This would be a typical daily program for a stroke patient:

1. Three to five periods in the physical therapy department.
    a. An individualized session with a physical therapist to exercise the involved limbs, keep the joints loose, strengthen muscles if possible, and teach the patient to use his limbs again.
    b. An ambulation class to teach walking.
    c. A mat class in which the patient learns to move his whole body again, exercises his trunk muscles, etc.
    d. A period of resistance exercises—if he is advanced enough, weights or special machines are used to strengthen muscles.
    e. Activities of daily living class where he learns such things as moving about in bed, getting in and out of bed, on and off the toilet, into the bathtub, how to wash, shave, dress and undress, and many other such things.
2. One or two periods in occupational therapy.
    Depending on his needs, the patient will work in the light functional, heavy functional, and/or homemaking sections of this department. Toward the end of his stay in the hospital, he may have a prevocational evaluation.
3. Speech therapy.
    For those patients with a speech disorder there is one period of therapy each day.

These represent the basic core of most patients' programs. In addition they may have regular or sporadic appointments with members of the staff from psychology, social service, or vocational counseling.

Periodically, usually once a month, the staff meets to review what progress the patient has made and to decide on changes in his program. At these meetings problems are discussed and plans for the future are made, including when the patient will be discharged and what he will do when he goes home.

34. What is the usual course of a stroke patient who is admitted for rehabilitation and how long does it take?

One thing both patient and family find difficult to accept is that progress after a stroke is always slow. Unless recovery takes place in the first two or three weeks one must measure progress in terms of weeks, months, and sometimes years. The average stroke patient stays in the hospital from two to four months but then may receive treatment for a number of months after discharge as an outpatient.

Usually he progresses in the following way. At first he is in a wheelchair most of the time, and he requires help dressing, getting in and out of bed, on and off the toilet, etc. In time he becomes able to propel his wheelchair himself, transfers alone, and feeds himself independently. In the meantime he has begun to walk in physical therapy. As his walking ability improves, he gradually abandons the wheelchair and begins to walk to his classes. His ability to care for himself slowly improves to the point where he becomes (more or less) completely independent, including bathing and dressing, which are difficult.

All of this can occur whether or not good function is regained in the hemiplegic arm. Of course, there is variation in the time and degree of accomplishment based on the severity of the stroke, the personality of the patient, the presence and severity of depression, and many other factors.

What has been described thus far is physical rehabilitation, and even that is heavily dependent upon the patient's personality and emotions. But total rehabilitation means much more than independence in walking and self-care.

It implies that the patient once more has a zest for living; that he has the desire and energy to do things, go places, and meet people. Herein lies the greatest challenge to rehabilitation medicine for, as anyone who has lived with a stroke patient knows, it is the rule for them to find it extremely difficult to do these things again. Guy Wint (author of *The Third Killer* and a stroke patient himself) said that everything looked gray to him, that things which interested and excited him before no longer did so. It was as if a damper had been put on all of life.

It is not known at this time whether anything can be done to help the patient go through this period or even to avoid it. Eventually most of them spontaneously emerge from the shadows. What we can do is understand what they are feeling and give them all the help and encouragement possible. Having a stroke is a lonely and terrifying experience; the feeling of isolation is intense. Those who are close to the patient can help by identifying with his feelings and letting him know that they understand.

35. Must one be content if the patient can only walk with a brace and cane?

In the final analysis the patient and the doctor must be governed in their attitudes and decisions by the realities of the patient's illness. This requires that they be neither pessimistic nor optimistic. Plans for the future, treatment prescriptions—all decisions should be based upon a clear evaluation of the situation and a projection into the future based on experience.

There are some patients who will walk only with a brace and cane. Usually it is a short brace (below the knee). Sometimes, after a year or two have passed, it may be discarded—but sometimes it may not.

Must one be content? It is doubtful if anyone is ever content in such circumstances, but one must adjust to them.

Would that our society could find a suitable middle ground where adjustment or contentment are concerned. There are some societies where people accept their circumstances without complaint even if they are very unfortunate. In societies like ours we have the opposite problem. Most of us have grown so accustomed to having everything we want we find it extremely difficult to adjust to deprivation.

Of course, it is better to walk without a brace or cane, but it may not always be possible.

36. Why are some patients able to walk at the rehabilitation center but not at home on weekends?

There are a few possible reasons for this. In the early months after a stroke the program at the hospital is like going to school. The patient wants to please the "teacher," but he or she has no interest in performing for the family at home. This is particularly true when walking is very difficult, as it always is at the beginning.

Another reason is that the patient may simply not be able to walk, again in the early stages, unless the therapist is there to prompt him. Walking is automatic for someone who is normal, but it is another thing when one must think of every movement before it is made. This is something which cannot really be understood unless it is experienced.

A third possible reason is that the patient may still be confused at times. This becomes obvious when his environment is changed. He is more settled and comfortable in the protected environment of the hospital while even his own home may represent insecurity.

37. When should a patient be treated as an inpatient and when as an outpatient?

This is variable, but there are some guidelines to go by. In general a person needs to be in the hospital or rehabilitation center during the early weeks after a stroke, if he does not recover fully in a short time. This is the period when he cannot walk safely and when he needs help with self-care and other day-to-day activities. Even at these times being in the hospital is not absolutely necessary, but it is advisable if rehabilitation facilities are available.

Suppose that a person lives in a rural area, the rehabilitation center is a hundred miles away, and it is financially or otherwise not possible for him to be hospitalized. This is the situation in which properly trained nurses can be of great help. Better yet, if the local hospital has a physical therapist on the staff, he and the nurses, under the direction of the physician, can do a great deal. True, it is not as desirable as being in a rehabilitation center, but the patient can do very well.

This is so because treatment in a hospital does not make the muscles start moving or sensation or speech return; these depend entirely upon natural healing. Treatment for stroke is to prevent complications, bring out all of the function which is there, teach the patient to live with his disability, and give support and encouragement. Under the right circumstances these things can be done in a community where there is no rehabilitation department or center.

When can the person be an outpatient? This is difficult to pinpoint. When he has made enough progress so that he doesn't need to use a wheelchair much of the time or at all, when he is practically independent in taking care of himself, and when his walking is quite safe, continuing treatment as an outpatient is feasible.

It is by no means necessary that he be completely rehabilitated before he goes home. As a matter of fact, there is a point where staying in the hospital is undesirable. Bear in mind that one of the goals of rehabilitation is to restore feelings of worth and independence. This may be ill served by keeping the patient in the hospital. Though he is not a child, it is a little like sending one off to school for the first time —we don't like to do it, but we know it's good for him. Actually, it is good practice in a rehabilitation center to have the patient go home on weekends shortly before he is discharged in preparation for being home full time. He then continues treatment as an outpatient if it is necessary.

38. How long should the patient be in rehabilitation treatment?

This is a highly individual matter and depends upon the severity of the stroke, the specific kinds of damage done, and the personality of the patient, to mention some of the more important factors. The doctor must make this decision and only he can do so.

Speaking generally, it is reasonable for a patient to remain in rehabilitation treatment as long as he continues to show measurable improvement. For example, let us suppose that Mr. Jones starts out with a completely paralyzed arm. Over a period of weeks he becomes able to move the whole arm but in slow stages. At first only the shoulder moves, followed by movement in the elbow, wrist, and fingers. All of these changes are recorded by the physical therapist who works to bring out as much function as possible.

If we suppose that he is a patient who does not recover fully, he eventually reaches a plateau, and the therapist no longer sees further improvement in the arm movements. The doctor, on his periodic examination, observes the same thing. This is the time to stop formal physical therapy for the arm, but it is extremely important that the patient and family be given exercises and activities to maintain whatever gains have been made.

Although it is sensible to discontinue treatment when the patient no longer shows measurable gains, it must be re-

181

membered that continued use of the affected limb can result in improved function. This part of the process can go on for many months after formal treatment is discontinued.

What has been said applies to all forms of rehabilitation therapy.

Unfortunately, but quite naturally, patients usually do not want to discontinue treatment unless they are fully recovered. They believe, again quite naturally, that as long as treatment continues there is the possibility of complete cure. If therapy for stroke were similar to an appendectomy for acute appendicitis, it would be reasonable to expect that treatment meant cure. Sadly, this is not the case. The return of function depends basically upon healing in the brain, and the doctor and therapist are nature's assistants—important to the process, but not the crucial factors.

But it is natural for the patient to react this way. Guy Wint, a man who had a stroke and wrote a book about it (see Appendix for full reference), said that even though he had decided he would not improve any further, one part of his mind continued to hope that he would and drove him to try every conceivable treatment he could find, including Chinese acupuncture and Hindu faith healing.

Although this is understandable for patients, those of us who live and work with them must keep a measure of balance and objectivity because important decisions are often based on whether or not treatment is continued.

It is obvious that this is a very difficult problem which requires understanding and courage on the part of those who are trying to help the patient. It is not good to sustain false hopes, for it postpones the time when the patient begins to adjust to his altered condition. Neither must he be told bluntly that there will be no further improvement. He needs to know the truth: that great improvement cannot be expected after a certain time, although he can continue to improve to a lesser degree over a long period of time.

It is difficult for family members and doctors, too, to tell the patient things he does not want to hear. This is where courage is needed. If these things are presented with understanding and compassion, they are usually accepted by the patient, and later he is grateful for having been told the truth.

39. Can a stroke patient be treated at home?

They can and often are treated at home. It is theoretically possible but rarely realistic to have all of the services at home which are available in a general hospital or rehabilitation center.

When circumstances dictate, doctors, nurses, and therapists can improvise and sometimes do very well. While it is not the same as operating on the kitchen table, it should be clear that one cannot duplicate the services of a hospital or rehabilitation center without a great deal of ingenuity, hard work, and expense.

40. Should someone who has had a stroke drive a car?

Some people who have had strokes can drive. Those who suffered mild strokes need no discussion; the question refers to patients who have had severe strokes.

Let us think for a moment about what is necessary to drive a car safely: arms and legs; good vision, hearing, judgment, and memory; the ability to read; and normal perception (as for depth, shapes, etc.). The last of these is very difficult to define but is just as important as the rest. Perception is discussed in detail in Question 1, Chapter 4.

Now let us consider how the person with a stroke may or may not qualify to drive. If one assumes the worst, one of his arms and one of his legs may be disabled for driving, but with a spinner on the steering wheel, automatic transmission, and proper training, this patient should be able to drive safely, assuming no other serious problems. In fact, poor function of an arm and leg is usually the least of the patient's problems.

A visual deficit is quite another matter. It will be recalled that the most common visual difficulty after a stroke is the loss of the peripheral field of vision on one side. The patient may have perfect vision when looking straight ahead but fails to see things "out of the corner of the eyes" on one side. Having never experienced this, it is difficult to imagine how disabling it can be and how dangerous in someone driving a car. Drivers depend more than they realize on the things which are seen in the peripheral visual fields. The loss of a field of vision on either side absolutely disqualifies a person for driving.

Except in rare circumstances hearing is not affected by a stroke so it need not be discussed here.

Unfortunately there are people without strokes who do not have good judgment. Forty thousand deaths and hundreds of thousands of injuries every year are proof of that fact. A stroke sometimes impairs judgment, temporarily or permanently, and if one has evidence that this is so, the patient should not be allowed to drive.

An adequate memory is not as important as the other factors mentioned. It may not prevent the person from the actual operation of an automobile, but it may make it very impractical if he cannot remember his way, rules of the road, and so forth.

Some patients with aphasia lose the ability to read and this, like poor memory, can make driving very problematic. The reasons are obvious.

Trouble with perception, that very subtle function of the mind that means so much without our being aware of it, can disqualify someone as a driver. This can best be illustrated by a true story.

During the first few months of his first trip out with the

driver-educator, a patient was instructed to stop at an inter-section. The traffic light at this intersection was located di-agonally across from where the car was stopped. The light changed, but the driver didn't move. When asked why, the patient stated that he didn't know whether he had the green or the red. In other words, three-dimensional objects looked flat to him. Of course, he probably could have figured out that the light on the left side faced him, but he was so con-fused at seeing a flat object where it should have been angu-lar that he became immobilized.

This is but one example of many different types of per-ceptual defects.

How then, does one determine whether or not a stroke pa-tient should drive? The first step is a careful physical examination by the doctor. This will turn up visual field de-fects, assess the function of the arms and legs, and give the doctor some idea of the patient's judgment, memory, ability to read, and so forth. Formal psychological and speech test-ing will provide explicit details about these same things. If examination and testing do not provide the answer one way or the other, then a trial of driving with a well-trained driver-educator will do so. A driving evaluation is a good thing for there are many patients who refuse to believe they cannot drive until they actually try it. Conversely, the person with only borderline difficulties is encouraged by the instructor to go through a period of training and often does so suc-cessfully.

Unfortunately, a history of many years of safe driving does not mean that someone will be able to drive after a stroke. However, many patients do drive after a stroke—sometimes better than they did before as a result of expert training.

It should not be assumed that any driving school can train a disabled person. This is a highly specialized field which calls for well-trained, experienced instructors and coordina-tion between doctor, psychologist, and instructor.

41. Can a patient take an air trip? What are the effects of high altitude?

Today's flying in pressurized cabins does not pose the problem that air travel did in bygone days.

The potential danger of high altitudes has to do with the fact that as one goes up the air pressure gets lower; this means that less oxygen is pushed through the lungs into the blood stream, and, as a result, less oxygen reaches the tissues of the body. For young, healthy individuals this is not a problem—they may become a little short of breath with exertion, but there is no danger. Older people or those who already have some trouble in the vascular system may not be able to tolerate the reduced amount of oxygen in the blood and can get into real trouble.

All of this is avoided in modern airplanes for the air pressure in the cabin is kept quite close to what it would be on the ground. There are minor changes in pressure which we feel in our ears and which cause us to swallow, but these are not dangerous. Of course, if one's inner ear passages are blocked there may be considerable pain, as many people know, but this is not a danger to life.

42. Where can I get help?

You may not realize it, but there are many people who are available to help you with your problems. This is probably truer if you live in a big city, but except for very isolated parts of the country there is considerable help available.

Throughout the course of the illness, but particularly at the beginning, your doctor is the best source of assistance. Immediately after the stroke has occurred he will see to it that the proper diagnostic studies are done and appropriate treatment given, either in or out of the hospital.

Rehabilitation

The fortunate patient will recover during the first month or two and after an additional period of recuperation can return to his previous life pattern.

For those who do not fully recover in a short time, one must immediately begin to think about rehabilitation. This is best accomplished in a rehabilitation center or in a large hospital with the appropriate facilities and staff. Almost all Veterans Administration hospitals have rehabilitation services. Your doctor will know if there are facilities in or near your community, and plans for admission should be made as soon as possible either as an inpatient or outpatient.

A good source of help at such times may be the doctor who is trained in rehabilitation medicine or physical medicine and rehabilitation (it is called by either name). If there is such a physician in your community, your doctor may want to seek his assistance. The two organizations representing this group of physicians are the American Academy of Physical Medicine and Rehabilitation and the American Congress of Rehabilitation Medicine; both are located at 30 N. Michigan Avenue, Chicago, Illinois, 60602. Professional people from other fields who are interested in the rehabilitation of disabled patients are also represented in the Congress.

If there are no rehabilitation facilities in your community, you must look to other sources. Visiting Nurse Associations can often provide help and sometimes have physical therapists on the staff. Both nurse and therapist, acting under a doctor's prescription, can be of considerable assistance when the patient comes home from the hospital and particularly if the patient has been at home from the beginning.

Your local health department may have nurses and therapists on the staff who are trained to give assistance and guidance in this type of problem. Community mental health programs should be kept in mind as sources of help for emotional problems.

The Easter Seal Society and the American Heart Association have literature on the subject and may have suggestions on where to find assistance.

An important Federal agency is the Social and Rehabilitation Service. It has representatives in almost every state through vocational rehabilitation agencies. Your local department of health can direct you to the nearest vocational rehabilitation office. They can provide financing for medical care, rehabilitation, job counseling, training in a new vocation, and other services for the patient who has the potential to return to work.

Every rehabilitation center has a large staff of social workers. It is an important part of the training of these workers to know what facilities are available in a community to help people who need it. If there is no rehabilitation center in your community, there is almost surely a social service agency to which you can turn. Incidentally, they are also trained to understand the multiplicity of problems which may arise with an illness such as stroke and can be a source of advice and guidance.

These and other organizations interested in the stroke patient are listed in the Appendix.

CHAPTER 6

Prognosis

1. Is the patient's life in danger?
2. Is it true that the first forty-eight hours are dangerous because the person can have another stroke?
3. Does the other half of the brain take over—is half of the brain a spare?
4. How long does it take brain cells to heal?
5. How soon after the stroke can you tell whether the patient will recover fully or not?
6. How long will the patient continue to get better?
7. Will the patient get worse?
8. Can a patient have a second stroke in later months or years?
9. Is there any difference between men and women with respect to recovery?
10. Does the age of the patient have anything to do with recovery?
11. If the patient is very emotional, does this slow down his recovery?
12. Is it foolish to hope for complete recovery?
13. Can the family do anything to speed recovery?
14. Will the patient recover faster at a rehabilitation center than at home?
15. Will the patient get any better after treatment is finished?

16. Should one lie to the patient to keep his spirits up?
17. When do you tell the patient he is not going to improve anymore?
18. If the patient is given a rest from treatment for a few months will he be able to come back and learn more?
19. Does stroke affect life expectancy?
20. What research is in progress on stroke?

Introduction

This chapter has to do with what one can expect in the long run after a stroke. Although this book is organized so that it can be read in any order, these questions should be kept for last since they require a knowledge of things which are explained in earlier chapters.

Most of the questions refer to people who do not recover fully from their strokes and will be of little interest to those who return to normal; these fortunate ones will not have to wrestle with the problems of learning to live with a disability —nor will their families.

Most of these questions, like those in the rest of the book, have been asked by the families of patients. They are the hardest questions to ask—and to answer.

1. Is the patient's life in danger?

By the time the reader has read this book, the danger to the patient's life will have passed. The dangerous time is immediately after onset, but then mostly in cases of hemorrhage rather than thrombosis or embolism.

We have already dealt with the question of a second stroke, which worries many people, but it is well to repeat that many things can be done to make this less likely. Weight reduction, treatment for high blood pressure, rest, exercise, better living habits, relief from tension—all these are important preventive measures.

2. Is it true that the first forty-eight hours are dangerous because the person can have another stroke?

This is not generally true. There are situations involving certain patients where it is true, but which patients these are and what is done to prevent a second attack is a complicated, technical matter that cannot be described here. The thing to remember is that in the majority of cases there is a single attack; many patients will go on to complete recovery, but even most of those who do not are quite safe from an immediate second episode.

Doctors are trained to recognize different types of stroke and know what can be done to prevent immediate recurrences. In most cases nothing has to be done, and nature begins the healing process promptly.

3. Does the other half of the brain take over— is half of the brain a spare?

Unfortunately, there is no evidence that either of these possibilities is true for people once the brain has developed. It appears to be true to some extent in the developing brains of children. For example, a child who is born with damage in the speech area may learn to speak because the other side of the brain takes over this function. However, this does not occur in adults. The other side is not a spare; by the time one reaches maturity it has assumed specific functions. If there were a part of the brain lying fallow, so to speak, then it could be available after a stroke, but nature did not design things that way.

There are people who have based methods of treatment on the theory that other parts of the brain take over after damage has occurred. There is no proof that this is true—on the contrary, the great body of experience that physicians have acquired through the years seems to point to the unfortunate fact that there are no spare parts in the brain.

4. How long does it take brain cells to heal?

It is difficult to answer this question categorically. Even doctors who study these matters cannot be absolutely sure. However, it is likely that the healing process is over in a few weeks. During this time the excess fluid gradually leaves the area around the damaged cells, and the mysterious process of healing within the cells begins to take place.

Often when people ask this question, they really want to know how long the patient will continue to get better, which is discussed in Question 6.

5. How soon after the stroke can you tell whether the patient will recover fully or not?

If the patient has not recovered fully by the end of the fourth week the odds are that he will not. However, he can get a great deal better, and this will not be known until many months later. This is true for most patients, but there are always exceptions to the general rule, and it is best to draw no conclusions until six or seven months have passed.

6. How long will the patient continue to get better?

One must be very specific about what is meant by getting better. Almost everyone means, how long will the arm or leg or speech get better.

To answer this as accurately as possible it is necessary to consider each part of the nervous system separately. Apparently, the healing of brain cells does not determine how long physical recovery will go on. Healing is over in a few weeks, but the patient may continue to develop strength in the arm and leg for seven to eight months. The same is true for sensation that has been lost on the hemiplegic side. This does not mean that everyone will recover completely in that time, but rather that one may see improvement for that long. After that the person may learn to use a partially disabled arm or leg better, but it is rare to see further actual recovery. However, it must be emphasized that the patient who is motivated to do so can continue to improve function in a limb long after the period of actual recovery has ceased.

One of our patients who had a stroke at the age of fifty-six ceased to have further return of function in the right arm and leg after the seventh month. He was able to walk and had roughly 50 percent return of function in the arm. Two years later he was working full time, going to a gymnasium every day where he swam for an hour and did calisthenics. As one sat and talked to him it was hard to believe that he had considerable residual disability in the arm and leg. On testing, his arm was as strong as a normal man's, although its movements were somewhat uncoordinated.

Turning to speech problems, which include all those discussed in Chapter 3, there are really two phases of recovery. It is during the first six months after a stroke that one will see very noticeable changes. The second period may extend for a number of years, but these improvements are much less dramatic. What this means is that beyond the healing of cells there must be a process of adjustment going on in the brain which we do not understand at all. Perhaps the most important adjustment is that which the patient and family make in learning to communicate with each other more effectively. It is sometimes amazing to see how well a husband and wife can converse when one of them is aphasic.

One woman said that the years after her husband's stroke were happy ones despite the fact that he was aphasic and could speak very few words. He developed a system of signs and she a sensitivity to what he was trying to say that was almost as effective as their previous means of communication. Perhaps misfortune had also drawn them closer together.

This sort of thing requires patience and persistence during the early months after a stroke; there must be an understanding normal speaker and a well-motivated patient.

The mental and emotional changes represent still another category. It will be recalled that there are a number of elements included in the designation "mental," such as memory, judgment, perception, and abstract thinking. These are very subtle and hard to measure. However, as one observes large numbers of patients over long periods of time they appear to continue to improve in these functions well into the second year after the stroke.

Emotional reactions represent a different problem because most of these do not result from changes in the brain but from the natural reaction of the patient to a serious and protracted illness. Depression, the most common reaction, often lasts for two or more years—not in every patient, but in many. There is great variation depending on the patient's personality, the severity of the stroke, the reactions of his family, and sometimes his social and financial status.

Visual problems may improve during the first six months but rarely show measurable changes after that.

7. Will the patient get worse?

In the great majority of cases, no! It depends upon what caused the stroke. If it was a thrombosis, as most of them are, the worst is over at the beginning, and the patient improves thereafter until he recovers completely or reaches a plateau.

If an unsuspected tumor is present, and this is very rare, the patient may get worse. This is always a warning and usually leads the physician to suspect a tumor if he did not before.

In certain cases where hemorrhage was the cause, there is a chance that the patient might become worse, but this can be anticipated and appropriate steps taken to halt the process.

It must be understood that one does not have a stroke unless there is fairly advanced trouble of some kind in the blood vessels. Therefore, the possibility of further difficulty always exists. However, a stroke seems to be a little like blowing off steam—blood pressure which was high returns to normal levels, tension and anxiety usually disappear, the patient is forced to rest, excess weight is often lost, he begins to exercise. It is for these reasons and others that are not yet understood that most patients do not continue to get worse after a stroke.

8. Can a patient have a second stroke in later months or years?

It is possible for patients to have a second stroke, but often they do not. There are a few reasons for this. In the preceding answer it was stated that having a stroke is like blowing off steam, the blood pressure usually returns to normal and the circumstances of the illness require the patient to rest, eat properly, lose weight, even exercise. Previously neglected conditions are properly cared for. In addition, the body constantly tries to improve unhealthy situations. If a portion of the brain is losing its blood supply, other vessels enlarge to bring more blood to the deprived area.

Of course, this idea cannot be carried to extremes. A stroke is usually the culmination of a process which has been going on for many years. One cannot expect that all of this will be reversed after the stroke. However, by paying attention to important things like rest, diet, exercise, and weight and by avoidance of tension, tobacco, and other excesses the chances for another stroke are diminished.

9. Is there any difference between men and women with respect to recovery?

Although there is a difference in the incidence of stroke in men and women (twice as many men have strokes as women), observation of many people with strokes does not show any sex difference in recovery. It is the severity of the basic cause and of the stroke itself which affect recovery.

10. Does the age of the patient have anything to do with recovery?

This is a "yes" and "no" answer. Basically, recovery is dependent upon the severity of damage to the brain: mild damage—good recovery; severe damage—poor recovery. However, this must be qualified since young people such as those with ruptured aneurysms obviously have greater powers of recuperation and greater energy. They usually work harder, and though they may be left with the same degree of disability as an elderly person, they may accomplish more and develop more function.

We recall a young man with a severe stroke involving the left side and blindness in the right eye who went on to law school after completing a rehabilitation program. Another young man who had just completed medical school when he had a stroke continued his specialty training, got married, and when last we heard from him had just become a father. Neither of these young men recovered completely from their strokes—both were left with reduced function in one arm and did not walk normally.

But age is not always a deterrent to good recovery. It is the mental attitude which is most important regardless of age.

11. If the patient is very emotional, does this slow down his recovery?

Before this question can be answered one must first define what is meant by recovery. It can be viewed in two ways. One can first talk about recovery in terms of the function of the arm and leg, the ability to speak if the patient is aphasic, the return of normal sensation, the recovery of normal vision. This kind of recovery depends upon how much the brain can heal itself, and it is *not* affected by emotionalism. It does not matter if the patient cries a lot or is depressed, angry, or very nervous. How much he recovers will depend primarily upon how much damage was done by the stroke and whether brain cells were destroyed or merely injured. In some cases cells are only injured and complete or nearly complete recovery takes place. In the rest, there is a combination of cells which are destroyed and those which are injured; recovery depends on the proportion of each. For example, if someone becomes almost but not quite normal again, it means that most of the cells in the area of the stroke were only damaged. If he is left with a great deal of weakness, aphasia, etc., it means that a large proportion of cells were destroyed.

Most people who ask this question, including both patients and their families, are referring to this physical type of recovery, and with very good reason. They want the patient to be normal again—to be the way he or she was before the stroke. Unfortunately, this cannot be in some patients and, therefore, one must talk about another kind of recovery.

The purpose of rehabilitation is to help bring about this

second kind of recovery. In this type the person who has had a stroke recovers his ability to do many or all of the things he did before despite residual weakness or other disabilities. He develops a satisfactory pattern of life even though it's not the same life he led before. He recovers a zest for living again, an interest in what is going on around him, a feeling that life is worth living despite the changed conditions. That type of recovery is very difficult to achieve, but to some extent it is in the hands of the patient, his family, and those who are trying to help him. But only to some extent, since the basic personality of the patient will be very important. If, for example, the patient was poorly adjusted to life before the stroke, it is not very reasonable to expect that he will be able to adjust any better after having an illness which leaves him with handicaps. Even here one must qualify, for there are some people who unconsciously welcome a stroke because of subconscious feelings of guilt and the desire to be punished. Leaving aside this kind of situation, it is possible for the person who was reasonably happy before his stroke to adjust to his changed condition. Many have done it.

In this type of recovery, emotionalism may be a deterrent. Specifically, depression, anger, and anxiety can slow down the process or keep it from happening at all. And this applies to the patient's family as well as to the patient himself.

For example, we recall a man who appeared to be accepting the fact that his left arm no longer functioned well, that he had to use a brace and cane for walking. He did so well that he returned to his job about five months after a very severe stroke. However, his wife, who was perfectly healthy, could not adjust to the changes in their lives and became so depressed that she often talked of suicide. Naturally, the man thought that all of this was his fault and became terribly unhappy.

In approaching this problem one must realize that it is

199

virtually impossible to change people's personalities. However, every attempt must be made to find the positive elements in the patient's makeup and help him to a better adjustment. Family members who react as did the wife described should seek psychiatric help.

Many times this question is asked because the patient tends to cry a lot, particularly in the early weeks or months after a stroke. This does no harm, and it does not always mean that he is depressed. It seems that the crying trigger in the brain is easily tripped after a stroke—some patients even cry in the midst of laughing. Eventually this wears off.

12. Is it foolish to hope for complete recovery?

That depends entirely on when one is hoping for it. It is not foolish the day after the stroke has occurred or two weeks later, no matter how severely stricken the patient is. If by the end of one month he has not yet begun to show signs of good recovery, the possibility of complete cure is unlikely. However, if at that time (one month) he is improving rapidly he may yet go on to complete recovery. The patient who has not fully recovered by six months will not do so, and it would be foolish then to hope for complete recovery.

All of this refers to physical recovery. The kind of recovery that is perhaps most important is that which permits the patient to live with some degree of contentment despite residual disabilities. It is never vain to hope for that—and one should never stop working for it.

13. Can the family do anything to speed recovery?

Once again, it depends on how recovery is defined. If it refers to return of function in the arm and leg, the family can do nothing to influence this process because that is between nature and the patient.

If, however, recovery is defined as that point at which

the disabled patient feels he is ready to pick up life where he left off before the stroke, the family may be able to help a great deal. Life will rarely be exactly as it was before—that is usually impossible, but many patients have a full and satisfying existence after a stroke.

In this aspect of recovery the family can be of tremendous help. They can understand the patient's turmoil in the early days, be patient with his explosions, try to lighten his depression by being cheerful themselves, help him to find new interests or rekindle old ones. If family members don't allow themselves to become depressed or anxious, they can shorten the time necessary for the patient's recovery.

14. Will the patient recover faster at a rehabilitation center than at home?

This cannot be answered categorically for there are many elements which contribute to recovery: the severity of the stroke, the personality of the patient, the strength and stability of his family, the opportunity for treatment, to name a few.

Let us suppose that a patient can receive treatment by well-trained doctors and therapists at home, is strongly motivated to recover, and has a relatively mild stroke. He may do very well without ever going to a rehabilitation center. By contrast, someone may have the best of treatment in a rehabilitation center and do very poorly in the long run.

Treatment is important, but it must be remembered that there are other factors which are just as important, and recovery may very well depend on these.

15. Will the patient get any better after treatment is finished?

Always! One can make a categorical statement about this for we have seen hundreds of patients return months and years after treatment is concluded, and they are always better, assuming they haven't had another illness.

A lady with severe aphasia returned two years after the completion of her treatment. At the time of discharge her communication ability was estimated to be about 25 percent normal. On examination we found that she had improved considerably in the interim and was even talking of opening a small shop for knitting materials.

One would logically expect this, for we believe that subtle changes go on in the brain long after the initial healing process is over. These changes do not produce dramatic improvement, but it is always noticeable. Occasionally, it is striking. The patient can always hope that he may be the lucky one.

Perhaps there is something more than luck involved, for these people are usually very active and determined individuals. They are the ones who plunge in and try to pick up where they left off before the stroke. Maybe this frame of mind has something to do with changes in the brain. Of course, this is only speculation, but there are so many things we do not understand about the brain and the "mind," that nothing is beyond the realm of possibility.

16. Should one lie to the patient to keep his spirits up?

It is shocking how often this is done—and it always fails. Lying to the patient is ostensibly done for his benefit; what it usually means is that the person who lies is protecting himself. He is avoiding the unpleasantness of the truth; trying to escape the responsibility of helping the patient struggle with reality; perhaps just sparing himself the sight and sound of a very unhappy loved one or patient.

The alternative to lying is not the bare, blunt presentation of facts. One sometimes hears of doctors who approach the family a week after the stroke and say with great finality "That's it, he'll never recover and you might as well get used to it!" No one can tell at that point how much the patient will recover or the quality of his recovery.

Let us assume for the moment that it is now one year since the patient had his stroke, and he is not fully recovered. It is entirely likely that he himself knows that he will not be cured completely. It is not reasonable or prudent to assure him at that point that he will be perfectly all right again. He must know the truth but at the same time must have the positive aspects of his situation emphasized.

But family members often say that if you take away hope you take away everything. That may be true for a moment, but most human beings are resilient. Eventually they are able to refocus and establish new goals. Of course this takes time, but if one continues to hide the truth it only postpones the day when the patient will begin the process of living with reality.

Is it really kindness to keep someone indefinitely in a state of unhappy ignorance? Or is it better to redirect his hope into realistic channels?

17. When do you tell the patient he is not going to improve anymore?

This is one of the most difficult questions we are called upon to answer because it is impossible to be a prophet. We know from experience that some patients never recover completely, but we also know that *improvement may occur slowly over a long period of time.*

The doctor should be the one to discuss this subject with the patient. He will introduce it at the appropriate time. Of course, many patients know after seven or eight months that they will not recover fully if they haven't by that time. The emphasis by friends and relatives should be positive, should be focused on helping the patient pick up where he left off despite remaining weakness or disability.

18. If the patient is given a rest from treatment for a few months will he be able to come back and learn more?

The whole question of treatment for the stroke patient is relatively new. It wasn't too many years ago that people who had strokes were simply accepted back into the family circle, if they were lucky enough to have one. When the family was more important than it is now, when it was the custom to have one or more of the older generation living in the house, when there might be household chores for these senior citizens to do, someone who had a stroke was more likely to fit into the scheme of things without rehabilitation. Today one is less liable to find this, and it is evident that changing social patterns have made rehabilitation necessary.

A second reason for the development of rehabilitation measures for the disabled is that doctors have become more sophisticated and realize their responsibility to such people as stroke patients. In addition, government, reflecting the wishes of the people, has concerned itself with these problems and supports research and treatment for things like heart disease, cancer, and stroke.

All of this means that it is now taken for granted that people must have rehabilitation treatment for stroke. But let us stop for a moment and think about treatment. This question asks if the patient will be able to come back and *learn* more after a rest from treatment. Just what is being done in treatment?

The chapter on rehabilitation goes into some detail on this subject, but this question can be answered in a general way. The goal of rehabilitation treatment is to find out exactly what the patient has retained and what he has lost in the way of physical and mental capacities—and to help him fully utilize that which he has left. It is true there is learning involved here, as when a person learns to do things with one hand because the other is disabled or learns to walk with a brace and cane. But there is a mistaken notion that a patient can always learn to use an arm again or walk as he did before the stroke regardless of the degree of weakness in the arm or leg. We wish that this were so—that by applying certain treatments one could stimulate muscles to function normally again or teach a person with aphasia to talk again. Unfortunately we cannot always do this, for recovery depends primarily on healing in the brain.

Recovery from stroke is not like teaching a child to walk or talk, where time and practice are the important factors. If this were so, all patients would recover completely simply by continuing treatment long enough. This is what many patients and their families believe and why so many want treatment to go on indefinitely. This is understandable, for neither the mind nor the heart wants to admit that recovery may not be complete.

And so, to answer this question, it must be said that returning for more treatment after a rest and after the patient has reached a plateau, let us say seven or eight months after a stroke, will not usually result in further progress. He is more likely to slowly improve by going about his business at home and trying to rebuild the patterns of his life which the stroke interrupted. To be sure, this is not an easy thing to do, but it is far more fruitful than continuing the quest for more treatment.

19. Does stroke affect life expectancy?

The stroke itself does not affect life expectancy. It is an episode which results from many other things which do influence length of life such as heredity, arteriosclerosis (hardening of the arteries), high blood pressure, overweight, tension, excessive use of tobacco, certain kinds of heart disease, and many others. In other words, these are the basic reasons for a stroke, and they also have a great deal to do with how long one lives.

There are occasional cases where the stroke does influence life expectancy, but in the majority it does not.

20. What research is in progress on stroke?

In Chapter 1 on the cause of stroke and Chapter 3 on speech disorders there were questions dealing with research. Research is going on in these and other areas, and more attention is being directed to this problem. The American Heart Association has just created a new council to promote research and knowledge about stroke, and, as is well known, the Federal government is heavily invested in the solution of this problem. Most of the large medical centers and medical schools in the United States have projects under study which bear on the question of stroke.

In addition to research on cause and prevention, many studies deal with the treatment of stroke, both in the acute phase and in the weeks and months which follow. The role of drugs is being investigated, of oxygen therapy, of better methods of physical therapy. New devices and braces are being developed and new methods of teaching the patient the many things he must learn are under study.

No one can predict what tomorrow will bring in the way of new discoveries, new treatments. That is the history of medicine, and there is no reason to believe that it will not continue in the same tradition. In the meantime, we must occupy ourselves with today's business, the only business that really counts.

Appendix

Associations and Agencies

American Academy of Physical Medicine and Rehabilitation, 30 North Michigan Avenue, Chicago, Illinois, 60602. *Professional organization of physicians who are specialists in rehabilitation medicine (physiatrists).*

American Congress of Rehabilitation Medicine, 30 North Michigan Avenue, Chicago, Illinois, 60602. *Professional organization of diverse professional disciplines interested in rehabilitation.*

American Heart Association, 44 East 23d Street, New York, New York, 10010. *Local offices in many parts of the United States.*

American Nurses' Association, 10 Columbus Circle, New York, New York, 10019.

American Occupational Therapy Association, 251 Park Avenue South, New York, New York, 10010.

American Physical Therapy Association, 1790 Broadway, New York, New York, 10019.

American Speech and Hearing Association, 9030 Old Georgetown Road, Washington, D.C., 20014.

Association of Rehabilitation Centers, 828 Davis Street, Evanston, Illinois, 60201.

National Society for Crippled Children and Adults, 2023 West Ogden Avenue, Chicago, Illinois, 60612. *Local offices in many parts of the United States.*

Social and Rehabilitation Service, Department of Health, Education and Welfare, Washington, D.C., 20025. *Address of your state agency can be obtained from county or state medical society.*

Visiting Nurse Association, 107 East 70th Street, New York, New York, 10021.

Suggested Reading

GENERAL INFORMATION ON STROKE

Strokes: A Guide for the Family, American Heart Association (Publication #EM204), 19 pages. Single copies available free from your local Heart Association.

Strike Back at Stroke, U.S. Public Health Service Publication #596. Available from Superintendent of Documents, U.S. Government Printing Office, Washington, D.C., 20402. Single copies available free from your local Heart Association.

Strokes, Irvine H. Page, M.D., Collier Books, New York, 1963.

Up and Around, American Heart Association (Publication #EM358). Single copies available free from your local Heart Association.

Do It Yourself Again: Self-Help Devices for the Stroke Patient, American Heart Association (Publication #EM360), 45 pages. Single copies available free from your local Heart Association.

Care of the Patient with a Stroke, Genevieve W. Smith, Springer Publishing Co., New York, 1967.

GENERAL INFORMATION ON APHASIA

Understanding Aphasia: A Guide for Family and Friends, Martha L. Taylor, Institute of Rehabilitation Medicine, New York University Medical Center, 400 East 34th Street, New York, New York, 10016.

Appendix

Aphasia and the Family, American Heart Association (Publication # EM359), 26 pages. Single copies available free from your local Heart Association.

An Adult Has Aphasia, Daniel R. Boone, The Interstate Printers and Publishers, Inc., Danville, Illinois.

Dysphasia: Professional Guidance for Family and Patient, McKenzie Buck, Prentice-Hall, Inc., Englewood Cliffs, N.J., 1968.

REHABILITATION

Physical Rehabilitation for Daily Living, Edith Buchwald, McGraw-Hill Book Company, New York, 1952.

Activities of Daily Living for Physical Rehabilitation, Edith Buchwald Lawton, McGraw-Hill Book Company, New York, 1962.

Homemaker Programs in the United States, U.S. Public Health Service Publication #928. Single copies available from Superintendent of Documents, U.S. Government Printing Office, Washington, D.C., 20402.

Aphasia Rehabilitation Manual and Therapy Kit, Martha L. Taylor and Morton M. Marks, McGraw-Hill Book Company, New York, 1959.

BOOKS WRITTEN BY PEOPLE WHO HAVE HAD STROKES

Episode: Report On the Accident in My Skull, Eric Hodgins, Atheneum Publishers, New York, 1964.

Stroke: A Diary of Recovery, Douglas Ritchie, Faber & Faber, Ltd., London, 1960.

The Third Killer: Meditations on a Stroke, Guy Wint, Abelard-Schuman, Limited, New York, 1967.

Index

210